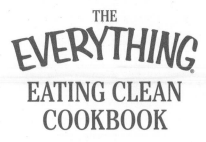

THE EVERYTHING EATING CLEAN COOKBOOK

Dear Reader,

We all strive to be healthy, fit, and live the best lives we possibly can. Yet busy days of full-time jobs, carpools, homework, deadlines, and household chores leave little spare time to prepare delicious, homemade, healthy meals, right? Wrong! I've compiled 300 recipes in this book that will show you how easy it can be to live a lifestyle that is nutritionally "clean," easy, and packed with fabulous foods that can keep you satisfied throughout the day.

As a busy mom, I know how hard it is to get everything done and still create delicious and nutritious meals! I am a certified personal trainer (CPT) and a certified fitness nutrition specialist (CFNS), but my "credentials" as a busy mom, athlete, and normal everyday person trying to live the healthiest life possible are just as important. That's why these recipes contain ingredients you can find at your local grocery store, and steps that are easy to follow. If you want you and your family to start eating healthier, you have to start somewhere. How about here? How about now?

I hope you enjoy these delightfully delectable meals as much as we do, and I wish you the best on your journey to a healthier you!

Sincerely,

Britt Brandon

Welcome to the EVERYTHING® Series!

These handy, accessible books give you all you need to tackle a difficult project, gain a new hobby, comprehend a fascinating topic, prepare for an exam, or even brush up on something you learned back in school but have since forgotten.

You can choose to read an Everything® book from cover to cover or just pick out the information you want from our four useful boxes: e-questions, e-facts, e-alerts, and e-ssentials.

We give you everything you need to know on the subject, but throw in a lot of fun stuff along the way, too.

We now have more than 400 Everything® books in print, spanning such wide-ranging categories as weddings, pregnancy, cooking, music instruction, foreign language, crafts, pets, New Age, and so much more. When you're done reading them all, you can finally say you know Everything®!

QUESTION

Answers to
common questions

FACT

Important snippets
of information

ALERT

Urgent
warnings

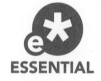

ESSENTIAL

Quick
handy tips

PUBLISHER Karen Cooper

DIRECTOR OF ACQUISITIONS AND INNOVATION Paula Munier

MANAGING EDITOR, EVERYTHING® SERIES Lisa Laing

COPY CHIEF Casey Ebert

ASSISTANT PRODUCTION EDITOR Jacob Erickson

ACQUISITIONS EDITOR Lisa Laing

DEVELOPMENT EDITOR Laura M. Daly

EDITORIAL ASSISTANT Ross Weisman

EVERYTHING® SERIES COVER DESIGNER Erin Alexander

LAYOUT DESIGNERS Colleen Cunningham, Elisabeth Lariviere, Ashley Vierra, Denise Wallace

Visit the entire Everything® series at *www.everything.com*

THE
EVERYTHING®
EATING CLEAN
COOKBOOK

INCLUDES:

Pumpkin Spice Smoothie • Garlic Chicken Stir-Fry
• Tex-Mex Tacos • Mediterranean Couscous •
Blueberry Almond Crumble . . . and hundreds more!

Britt Brandon, CFNS, CPT

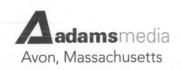
adamsmedia
Avon, Massachusetts

*To my wonderful husband, Jimmy, and my beautiful children,
Lilly, Lonni, and our newest on the way: I have you to thank
for making my life an absolute dream come true and for
showing me the true meaning of life every single day!*

An Everything® Series Book.
Everything® and everything.com® are registered trademarks of F+W Media, Inc.

Published by Adams Media, a division of F+W Media, Inc.
57 Littlefield Street, Avon, MA 02322 U.S.A.
www.adamsmedia.com

ISBN 10: 1-4405-2999-X
ISBN 13: 978-1-4405-2999-3
eISBN 10: 1-4405-3021-1
eISBN 13: 978-1-4405-3021-0

Printed in the United States of America.

10 9 8 7 6 5 4

Library of Congress Cataloging-in-Publication Data
is available from the publisher.

The information in this book should not be used for diagnosing or treating any health problem. Not all diet and exercise plans suit everyone. You should always consult a trained medical professional before starting a diet, taking any form of medication, or embarking on any fitness or weight-training program. The author and publisher disclaim any liability arising directly or indirectly from the use of this book.

Many of the designations used by manufacturers and sellers to distinguish their products are claimed as trademarks. Where those designations appear in this book and Adams Media was aware of a trademark claim, the designations have been printed with initial capital letters.

Nutritional statistics by Nicole Cormier, RD.

*This book is available at quantity discounts for bulk purchases.
For information, please call 1-800-289-0963.*

Contents

Acknowledgments

I would like to thank, first and foremost, Lisa Laing, my editor at Adams Media, for being the best teacher, having faith in me, and giving me this incredible opportunity.

Thank you to all of my wonderful family members who have been so supportive and proud throughout this process. Special thanks to my mom for showing me the importance of faith; my dad for teaching me to never give up; my "Miss Pam" for always being positive and honest; and my brother, Neal, for being my absolute favorite training partner and most challenging competitor yet.

To my amazing husband, Jimmy, who is my best friend, my biggest supporter, and the absolute love of my life: Your unwavering support and faith in me to achieve my dreams makes me love you even more! Thank you for taste-testing everything over all of these years . . . and being wonderfully honest. I love you so much and feel lucky to be by your side each and every day through this wonderful life we've built together!

And, for my amazing children, Lilly, Lonni, and our newest little one on the way, I thank you for absolutely everything and, yet, could never thank you enough! You make me want to be a better person, to strive to be the best I can be every day, and you are my daily reminder that life is a blessing to never be taken for granted. You have given me a better understanding of what is truly important in life, a different perspective on the world I hope to never lose, and a love that I can compare to nothing else. I love you more than anything, and I thank you for making life more amazing, each and every day!

Thank you! Thank you! Thank you!

Introduction

THE STANDARD AMERICAN DIET (perhaps appropriately known by its acronym, "SAD") is turning the United States into one of the unhealthiest nations in the world. Children, young adults, mature adults, and the elderly are all suffering the consequences of poor diets packed with dangerous preservatives, sugars, sodium, and synthetic additives created to preserve and prolong shelf lives and improve taste with minimized expenses. With the prevalence of fast-food options like prepackaged frozen meals, to-go boxes, and drive-through bags that cut time and offer on-the-go alternatives, the average American consumer receives little quality nutrition and rarely, if ever, consumes fresh ingredients.

Skipping breakfast, or not eating at all until dinner, has become the norm for many: A fast-food sandwich is considered "balanced" because it has meat, lettuce, tomato, cheese, and a bun, and a weeknight dinner that requires little more than peeling back a film and popping it into a microwave oven has become commonplace in households across America. While quick and easy, the dangers from these diets are never-ending and extremely unhealthy, and that's exactly what the "clean" lifestyle strives to simplify.

It's time to get back to basics . . . literally! One of the main issues that plague America's health is the overwhelming amount of processed ingredients in the foods that make up the daily diet. When looking at a package of candy, a batch of fast-food fries, or a meal served from a microwave-safe package, it's hard to determine the origins of the ingredients or how these "foods" were produced. Conversely, by looking at a salad, a grilled fillet of fish, or a plate of stir-fried vegetables, it's quite easy to determine where the ingredients came from. Put simply, this is the goal of clean eating: to eat foods that can be easily traced back to their origins in nature.

In order to function properly, the body requires proper nutrition from the vitamins, minerals, and nutrients derived from the proteins, carbohydrates, and fats in the foods we eat. In order to function *optimally*, these valuable nutrients should come from clean foods that are natural, fresh, and as minimally processed as possible. Clean eating provides the body with all the nutrition it needs for use in whichever way it needs it . . . the way it was designed to. Simplifying the foods you ingest simplifies the digestion process and maximizes their benefits. Simplicity at its best!

Returning your body, your mind, and your life to a naturally healthy state is a lot easier than it sounds. The clean lifestyle is just that—a lifestyle. Clean eating is not only simple, easy to understand, easy to apply to everyday life, and packed with foods that leave you satisfied—it also gets you on track to having the healthiest body, mind, and life possible! You can improve almost every aspect of your life just through diet. When you eat clean, you'll improve your energy levels, ability to focus, stress levels, quality of sleep, athletic stamina, and the overall condition of your entire body. Once you reap the rewards of a clean lifestyle, you wouldn't dream of returning to your old, poor lifestyle choices that left you drained of energy, mental clarity, and zeal for life. Your body will be the well-designed machine you have always dreamed of.

Look for tips and suggestions throughout this book to help you plan ahead, create meal plans, write out shopping lists, swap hazardous ingredients for healthy alternatives, and streamline preparations. You'll also find recipes for your family's favorite comfort foods like delicious breakfast muffins and creamy dinner dishes made the healthy, clean way!

While many people credit their lack of exercise and poor diet to a lack of time, the truth is that optimizing your body's condition doesn't have to be time-consuming at all. You won't have to make any sacrifices (except for the time you spent in the drive-through) when you switch to a cleaner lifestyle. Creating delicious home-cooked meals that are packed with fresh ingredients and healthier alternatives can be as efficient as any other option.

Millions of people have enjoyed the amazing and plentiful benefits of living a clean lifestyle. Are you ready to be one of them?

CHAPTER 1

The Clean Eating Lifestyle . . . Simplified

Congratulations! You've made the decision to become more informed and educated about living your healthiest life. The clean lifestyle helps you to take control of your health and move toward positive improvements like increased energy levels, better focus, fewer illnesses, and more vitality. This cookbook will be your guide to the life-changing benefits of "eating clean." This is not a diet—it's a complete change in the way you eat. You'll explore the many satisfying ways to enjoy whole, unprocessed, natural foods every day—one meal at a time. And after only a few weeks, you'll start to reap the health benefits of eating clean.

The Origins of Clean Eating

While many generations, movements, and individuals take credit for playing a major role in bringing clean eating to the world, the truth is that clean eating has its roots in every culture that appreciates food, the earth, and the human body. It's believed that the clean eating movement began in the United States in the early 1960s by people in search of natural products and natural foods that would be as beneficial for them as they would be for the planet. The original goals were to consume foods in the forms closest to their natural states, eliminating toxic substances found in man-made ingredients, while conserving natural resources by taking only what was needed and giving back by composting, planting new crops, and starting another growing cycle.

The clean lifestyle has undergone changes and improvements over the years as new health information became available, but it still holds the same original goals and beliefs today as it did at its inception. We know even more now about the importance of a diet consisting of fresh fruits and vegetables, lean meats, and whole grains than we did ten, twenty, or fifty years ago. We've learned about the dangerous effects of sugars, certain fats, refined products, excessive salt, and many other ingredients (synthetic and otherwise) when consumed in excess. According to countless studies, removing these ingredients from your diet will help to prevent illness and disease while improving your health and vitality.

Clean Eating Basics

The key points of clean eating are simple to apply to everyday life once you understand them and why they're important.

If You Can't Get It from Nature, You Shouldn't Eat It

This is the basis of the entire eating clean lifestyle. Think about it: There is no such thing as a Twinkie tree or a potato chip bush. Your main goal is to eat foods as close to their natural state as possible. This is the easiest guide to what foods should and shouldn't be included in your clean daily meals. Even foods that may *seem* like healthy options—like fruit juices and dried fruit—can be sugary pitfalls that lack the full nutrition available in the actual whole fresh fruits.

Consuming natural whole foods helps you get the maximum benefit from every calorie consumed. There is a major nutritional difference between 200 empty calories from a cookie, a slice of cake, or a handful of processed potato chips and 200 calories of fresh fruits, colorful veggies, or lean protein. By sticking to natural foods, you can make sure that you're getting the most out of every bite.

FACT

While the manufacturers of certain produce pesticides stand by their products' safety, certain chemical compounds used to combat bugs and preserve produce have been suspected in contributing to health issues in consumers. From attention-deficit disorders to severe illnesses like cancer, pesticides may or may not play a role; the best bet is to purchase organic, pesticide-free produce.

Eat Five or Six Meals Every Day

Most people scratch their heads at the concept of eating often. You may think that three square meals a day is the healthiest way to eat, or that more food equals more fat. However, research has shown that smaller, more frequent meals benefit the body far more than the archaic "three meals a day" plan. Spreading your daily calories out between five to six meals and snacks every two to three hours plays a major role in the clean lifestyle. Smaller, more frequent meals reduce hunger, provide constant fuel for your body, and limit excess calories that would be otherwise stored as fat.

Think about Future Activity Before Eating

Having a good idea about your activity for the hours following your meal can help you decide what's best to eat. If you're looking forward to an intense workout, prepare a more energy-boosting meal than you would if you were going to spend the next couple of hours sitting in front of a computer at an office desk. By thinking about the activities you'll engage in for the three hours between meals, you can better gauge the components of your meal or snack.

Pay Attention to Fats

Contrary to the fad diets limiting fats, promoting fats, or cutting them out all together, clean eating has made one point simple: Stick to the "good" fats. An easy rule of thumb is to eat the "un" fats: monounsaturated fats and polyunsaturated fats. These two types of fats, usually found in fish, nuts, and healthy oils, are heart healthy and brain healthy.

QUESTION

Is chocolate part of a "clean" lifestyle?
Loaded with sugar, milk, calories, and fat, chocolate does not fit the guidelines of the clean lifestyle in any way, shape, or form. Some great alternatives to chocolate are available, such as carob and emulsified dates, and using these substitutes can allow you to enjoy chocolaty-tasting treats without actually consuming chocolate. Or, try using baking chocolate, which has less milk and fat—as in the Best-Ever Cocoa Caffe Brownies in Chapter 13.

Saturated fats and trans fats are the no-no's to avoid. Saturated fats morph from solids at room temperature to liquids when heated, like butter. These fats have been directly linked to increasing the levels of "bad" cholesterol (LDL) in the blood. Trans fats (a.k.a. "partially hydrogenated oils") are added to certain foods as an inexpensive way to increase shelf life, eliminate the need to refrigerate, and improve the taste of fast foods and fried foods.

Relearn What a Real Portion Is

Because everything in the Standard American Diet is supersized, all-you-can-eat, or available in bottomless bags and boxes, the average person has completely forgotten, or never truly understood, what a single serving is. As you transition to the eating clean lifestyle, it's important to pay attention to the type and amount of foods you consume; this can easily be done by becoming familiar with what a true serving is for each type of food.

- **Dairy:** 1 serving is equal to 1 cup of milk or yogurt, 1 ounce of cheese
- **Meat:** 1 serving is equal to 3 ounces of protein like fish, chicken, or beef; comparable to the size of your fist or a deck of playing cards

- **Vegetables:** 1 serving is equal to 1 cup of raw leafy greens, or about the size of your fist; ½ cup cooked vegetables, or about the size of a deck of cards
- **Fruits:** 1 serving is equal to 1 medium-sized fruit the size of a tennis ball, or ½ cup sliced fruit

Avoid Processed Sugars and Sweeteners

Refined sugars are everywhere! When eating clean, you should avoid sodas, white sugar, sugary snacks and treats, and even the artificial sweeteners labeled "natural." Recent research done on the effects of refined sugars on the blood, brain, and body shows that this one culprit can cause blood sugar spikes and crashes that result in fatigue, lack of focus, compromised immune systems, and serious diseases like type 2 diabetes.

One of the best parts of the clean lifestyle is that you can instead sweeten your breakfasts, baked goods, and delectable desserts with healthier alternatives. The natural sweeteners well known in clean lifestyle nutrition are highly recommended over refined sugars because they are processed as little as possible. The most popular unrefined sweeteners are Rapadura, Sucanat, and agave nectar, with more hitting the market every year. While they may be difficult to find at your local grocery store, any health food store will provide you with a wide selection of unrefined natural sweeteners such as these.

Avoid Processed Dairy

When living the clean lifestyle, you want to drink very little, if any, cow's milk. Why? First, there are so many steps necessary to pasteurize and prepare cow's milk for safe consumption. Second, consider the lengthy list of antibiotics, hormones, and steroids administered to most milked livestock—they're not clean items. While many feel that soy milk may be a healthier alternative to cow's milk, there has been much debate about the consequences of consuming soy products due to the higher levels of estrogen found in them.

A simple, clean substitute for cow's milk and soy milk is almond milk, a product of simply emulsified almonds combined with water and few other ingredients. This low-sugar option can be a delicious and smooth-textured milk alternative that tastes quite similar, yet has much more natural ingredients that require far less processing or added ingredients. You can find almond milk at most regular grocery stores.

Combine Complex Carbohydrates, Lean Protein, and Healthy Fats at Every Meal

Not only does this concept allow for delicious variety at each and every meal, but it ensures that your body always has the fuel it needs for any job it needs to do. Whether you're gearing up for an intense workout, preparing for a long day, or taking it easy after some strenuous activities, your body utilizes the combinations of carbohydrates, proteins, and fats in order to fuel, endure, or recover properly. By eating a combination of these three types of foods, you can be sure that you're giving your body the adequate nutrition it needs . . . all the time.

Avoid Alcohol

Packed with empty calories, alcohol can be a major pitfall of any diet. Alcohol has nothing healthy to contribute and only makes your body's systems work harder to detoxify your body. You should minimize your alcohol intake or avoid it altogether in order to promote optimum health. If you're going to partake in a treat, indulge in something special that won't unravel all the good you've done for your body and your life. A recipe from this book for a delicious smoothie, delectable baked good, or creamy dish will be far more rewarding and satisfying than one drink . . . and you can still feel good about your choices the next morning.

Drink Lots of Water

It sounds simple, but most people don't drink the recommended eight 8-ounce glasses of water per day. In order to function properly, your body (which is made up of mostly water) has to have water. Water is your best friend—it eliminates toxins, satisfies fake hunger pains, and abolishes dehydration. Some devout soda drinkers have lost significant amounts of weight just by cutting out soda and drinking water instead.

If you already drink a ton of water, great! If not, the simplest way to increase your water consumption is to slowly replace your sugary beverages with water. Instead of a glass of juice in the morning, you could have water. Instead of the can of soda in the afternoon, drink some water. If the plain taste of water is what halts your consumption, try flavoring your water with a squeeze of citrus like lemon, lime, grapefruit, or orange.

ESSENTIAL

Comparisons between tap water and filtered water have shown dramatic differences in levels of certain minerals and chemicals that may, or may not, contribute to health issues. By drinking filtered water, you can be sure that you're ingesting fewer chemicals and toxins, thus maintaining a cleaner environment inside and out.

Build a Clean-Eating Family

If you're thinking that the hardest part of making the switch to a cleaner diet will be getting your family on board, have no fear. Many people find it difficult to transition from traditional fatty foods made with undesirable ingredients to a cleaner variety, but more often than not, the hesitance is more psychological (about the change) than physical (about the taste). Breaking through the resistance to cleaner foods can easily be done by preparing delicious meals that appeal to your family's tastes, yet include more natural ingredients. The recipes in this book cater to "normal" tastes by using fresh, natural ingredients to compose the everyday favorites we all know and love.

The clean lifestyle is one that has profound effects that last a lifetime, and this is important to convey to anyone who may not be on board with cleaner eating. The clean eating lifestyle can lead to a more active, enjoyable lifetime free of health issues and setbacks caused by foods that may have toxic ingredients. Simple, fun activities like building your own organic garden and exploring the "eat the rainbow" mentality (of eating a fruit or veggie in each color of the rainbow every day) can help you get your kids on board and create a feeling of joint effort in the transition to a cleaner lifestyle. By teaching children and adults the importance and benefits of cleaner eating, the lifestyle can be easier to accept by even the most steadfast resister out there!

Benefits of the "No Diet" Way of Life

Although eating clean foods promotes the healthiest functioning of all your body's systems, the benefits are much more significant than just an improvement in how you feel. Following are some of the other benefits you'll enjoy.

Faster Metabolism

Consuming smaller meals every two or three hours provides your body with constant fuel. This eating schedule solves the most common issue dieters experience: not feeling full after meals. With clean eating, your hunger and cravings are satisfied by the smaller doses of delicious foods, *and* you get to increase the number of times you eat to six! By eating every two or three hours, your body doesn't end up running out of gas. When people go very long periods without eating (hours, or even an entire day), they suffer from fatigue, and lack of mental focus—both of which are serious consequences resulting from frequent blood sugar drops, etc.

By eating smaller meals six times a day, your metabolism speeds up because your body is always utilizing the available complex carbohydrates, proteins, and healthy fats as fuel instead of storing them in preparation for another long stretch without. Using energy instead of storing it means that you'll be able to reduce your body fat while increasing lean body mass.

Improved Brain Function

When clean foods replace the toxic, nutrient-lacking foods in your brain, some of the first noticeable improvements you'll see are in energy levels and mental clarity. "Unclean" foods come with long ingredient lists of hard-to-pronounce names, provide little or no natural substance, and are lacking in vital vitamins and nutrients. They also cause fluctuating hormone and blood sugar levels, and offer little in the way of nutrition that promotes vitality.

The good news is that by replacing the poor foods that wreak havoc on the body's systems with natural whole foods that deliver proper nutrition on a regular basis, all of the body's systems can be back on track with peak performance in no time! That means more energy, less fatigue and sluggishness, better ability to focus, and improved memory and brain functioning . . . and who wouldn't want all that?

Improved Performance and Recovery

Although performance and recovery may seem to be important only to athletes, fitness enthusiasts, and bodybuilders, the body's ability to perform at its finest and recover most efficiently should matter to everyone. Whether you are training for a triathlon or just taking leisurely walks with your dog every day, your body needs to be able to have the right nutrition to perform tasks when called upon, and then fully recover following an activity in preparation for the next. The right nutrition to fuel performance and recovery is a combination of complex carbohydrates, lean proteins, and fats. The clean lifestyle promotes a combination of these three foods at every meal, so your body always has the right nutrients available when needed without having to plan.

Better Hydration

Water is a constant multitasker in the body. Acting as a detoxification specialist, the ultimate clean fuel, and a refreshing comfort to everything from the organs to the skin, water plays an intricate part in the clean lifestyle. Flushing out the toxins that remain from all of the poor ingredients consumed is extremely important to getting your body back on the right track.

Replacing sugary drinks and sodas with water is one of the most significant steps you can make toward cleaning up your diet and your health. With constant hydration, your body will no longer suffer from dehydration headaches, fatigue, and those fake hunger pains that make you reach for a sugary snack instead of a glass of water. Last, but certainly not least, water has no calories, so it doesn't matter how much you drink . . . your body can only shed excess weight rather than gain it!

Getting Started: Prep Your Kitchen

In order to create the best possible food combinations, and have them readily available for main meals, snacks, and on-the-fly situations, getting your kitchen in tip-top shape is priority #1. You'll just need a few inexpensive basics—most of which you probably already own—to craft anything from delicious soups and salads to beautiful entrées and delectable desserts. Here is a simple checklist to make sure you're ready to go.

Assorted Knives

Cutting, chopping, peeling, and dicing can be made easier with a good set of sharp knives. Not only will good knives make for faster food prep, but your hands won't suffer from having to work harder to compensate for dull, inappropriate knives.

Cutting Boards

Cutting boards can contain messes and make cleanup easier, making them a definite necessity. Whatever you feel most comfortable with, wood or glass, is what makes a cutting board right for you. Make sure it's small or large enough to fit in your prep space, and always be sure that you clean your boards thoroughly to prevent cross-flavor contamination.

ALERT

Even though they may be cheaper, plastic and silicone cutting boards can be problematic. Porous materials such as these (and wood boards) can absorb food juices, smells, and tastes from meats and produce, lending those tastes to foods prepped later on the same board. Also, plastics can sometimes contain dangerous chemicals that can be toxic if they seep into your food. Repeated washing and heating (in the dishwasher) can contribute to releasing those toxins. Better to just spend the extra dollar and get a glass board.

Storage Containers

Storage containers are a must for any clean eater because they can keep prepared meats, vegetables, grains, and fruits perfectly fresh and ready to go whenever you need them. Consider getting glass containers—they are heavier but do not retain the smell and taste of other foods stored in them.

Emulsifier

Costing only a few dollars, this important tool can transform a tedious job of mashing or puréeing into a simple, quick, and easy task. Soups, sauces, and purées take only minutes with this handy tool, and confine cleanup to only one item! Available at almost any store, an emulsifier is a hand-held blender that can be submerged into liquid or softened solids (like boiled potatoes or cooked legumes) and emulsify the contents quickly and easily, needing only a quick rinse with soap and water before returning to its drawer.

Food Processor or Chopper

Cutting boards make for a great spot to do smaller jobs, but a food processor can perform the same job on a larger scale in a tenth of the time. A little pricier than a handheld chopper, a food processor can be purchased with a large or small capacity, and can make food prep a breeze.

Scale and Measuring Cups and Spoons

Relearning portion sizes will come naturally . . . after practice. In the meantime, rely on measuring cups and a kitchen scale. They are inexpensive, easy to use, and simple to store.

Notebook

Although completely optional, a kitchen notebook can help you keep track of anything of meaning to you. Maybe you found an ingredient you like (or don't), noticed you normally overestimate a certain food, figured out a new favorite recipe . . . whatever the case may be. This notebook may become your best ally in revamping your diet and your life!

The Best (and Worst!) Ingredients

Here are the most common, and delicious, clean foods available in each category of protein, carbohydrates, and fats. While these lists are not all-inclusive or complete, they are great introductions to the clean ingredients and whole foods you'll be using every day. You may find that you already include many or most of these recommended foods in your daily diet. Most of the recipes that follow include these foods.

CLEAN PROTEINS: LEAN MEATS, SEAFOOD, AND BEANS

- beans (all, in natural forms)
- raw nuts and seeds
- natural nut butters
- lean beef cuts
- chicken breasts
- fish (fresh)
- shrimp
- lean turkey breast (ground or whole)
- pork tenderloin
- eggs
- fat-free plain yogurt (regular or Greek-style)
- low-fat cottage cheese
- non-dairy milks (almond, rice, and soy)
- kefir
- tofu
- tempeh
- quinoa, hemp seed, and flax seeds (considered proteins and carbohydrates)

CLEAN COMPLEX CARBOHYDRATES: WHOLE GRAINS

- bran cereal
- rolled oats
- cream of wheat
- buckwheat
- 100 percent whole wheat bread
- sprouted grain bread
- 100 percent whole wheat pasta
- 100 percent whole wheat tortillas
- bulgur
- quinoa
- millet
- wheat germ

CLEAN COMPLEX CARBOHYDRATES: VEGETABLES

- beets
- broccoli
- cauliflower
- carrots
- celery
- onions
- peppers
- green beans
- peas
- corn
- potatoes
- sweet potatoes
- spinach
- cabbage
- kale
- romaine lettuce
- zucchini
- squash

CLEAN COMPLEX CARBOHYDRATES: FRUITS

- avocado
- mango
- papayas
- apples
- bananas
- blueberries
- strawberries
- blackberries
- raspberries
- oranges
- grapefruit
- pineapple
- lemons
- limes
- grapes
- kiwi
- cantaloupe
- honeydew melons
- pears
- peaches
- pomegranates
- tomatoes

CLEAN FATS

- olive oil
- canola oil
- coconut oil
- avocado oil
- almonds
- pistachios
- cashews
- walnuts
- flaxseeds
- hemp seeds
- fatty coldwater fish

CLEAN SWEETENERS

- agave nectar
- bee pollen
- organic honey
- fruit sugar
- Sucanat
- Rapadura

The Worst Offenders: Non-Clean Ingredients

- White sugar
- Brown sugar
- Artificial sweeteners
- "Natural" artificial sweeteners
- White flour
- "Refined" ingredients
- Fatty cuts of meat
- Solid oils

Helpful Tips and Suggestions

While the clean eating lifestyle will create amazing changes in how your brain, body, and life functions, you may occasionally get feelings of nostalgia for your old ways. Once the clean lifestyle takes hold and works its magic, the difference will be obvious when you veer off-track with some not-so-clean foods. The sluggish feelings, mental fog, and lack of energy can flood back with just a couple of indulgent meals . . . and all of these feelings will remind you why you were searching for a cleaner lifestyle to begin with. It can seem frustrating and uncomfortable to feel at all restricted, to be tempted by poor foods, or to feel like you've just run out of new ideas to keep things interesting, especially in the beginning when you're getting into the swing of the clean lifestyle. In order to keep everything moving in a positive direction and on the right track to optimal health, here are some helpful tips and suggestions.

- **Don't Keep Poor Foods Around:** At home, at work, or on the run, avoid keeping empty foods as available options. Resist temptation by removing the temptation.
- **Pack It Up:** Prepare meals and snacks at home and bring them along when you're out for the day. That way, you'll never need to turn to fast food or takeout.
- **Plan Ahead:** You can create an entire week's meal plan around your favorite recipes (and those you plan to try out). By knowing the meals that you plan to make, you can anticipate what ingredients you'll need, and you'll find pleasure in looking forward to certain meals. Taking the time to sit down and relax on a Sunday (or whatever day you choose) and focus on what foods you'd like to have and create a week's meal plan will take the guesswork out of mealtimes and save time and energy.
- **Prep Ahead:** Hand-in-hand with creating a meal plan for the week is the timesaving concept of preparing ingredients ahead of time. If you know you'll be using diced onions, chopped zucchini, or sautéed chicken in your upcoming recipes, you can prepare them ahead of time and store them in separate storage containers for specific meals. This is a major timesaver and daily simplifier in the clean eating lifestyle.
- **Shop Smart:** Many people fear that eating natural, whole foods means more expensive shopping trips, but this is not at all true. By shopping smart, you can spend the same amount (and even less!) on clean foods than you would on poor foods. Creating meal plans based on the items on sale at your local grocery store can make eating clean very inexpensive. Certain lean meats, seafood, vegetables, and fruits are discounted at certain times of the year or on weekly rotations; by stocking up on frozen meats on sale and using the fresh seafood and produce that's on sale for the week, you can provide for an entire week in one shopping trip, save money, and waste less.

- **Keep Water on Hand . . . at All Times:** No matter where you're going or what you plan on doing, make sure you have plenty of water with you. If you have it available, you'll be more likely to drink it. Rather than having to stop for a drink at the convenience store (and be tempted by whatever else may be sold there), you'll have planned ahead, prepared ahead, and saved yourself the time, trouble, and temptation. That's success!

CHAPTER 2

Breakfasts

Fruity Egg White Frittata

This delicious blend of fruit atop a light and fluffy egg white frittata makes a surprisingly sweet breakfast treat. Light, but packed full of protein, this breakfast will rev up your day without weighing you down.

INGREDIENTS | SERVES 6

1 cup sliced strawberries

1 cup blueberries

1 cup raspberries

10 egg whites

1 teaspoon vanilla extract

1 tablespoon agave nectar

Essential Vanilla Extract

When a recipe calls for vanilla, use *real* vanilla extract. Although real vanilla extract is more expensive than imitation, the flavor is far superior. Store it in a cool, dark place.

1. Preheat oven to 350°F and spray an oven-safe frying pan with olive oil cooking spray.

2. Over medium heat, sauté all fruit together until lightly heated and softened.

3. While fruit is heating, whisk together the egg whites, vanilla, and agave nectar briskly until well blended. Add to the frying pan, covering fruit completely.

4. Continue cooking until the center solidifies slightly and bubbles begin to appear.

5. Remove from heat and place into preheated oven.

6. Cook for 10–15 minutes, or until frittata is firm in the center.

PER SERVING Calories: 70 | Fat: 0.5 g | Protein: 6.5 g | Sodium: 92 mg | Fiber: 2.5 g | Carbohydrates: 11 g | Sugar: 7.5 g

Turkey, Egg White, and Hash Brown Bake

You can beat any craving for a hearty but healthy breakfast with this satisfying dish. Combining delicious ground turkey breast and hash brown potatoes in a one-pot dish, this is a great meal for breakfast or any other time of day.

INGREDIENTS | SERVES 16

1 pound ground turkey breast, browned
1 pound shredded potatoes
16 egg whites
4 whole eggs
2 teaspoons all-natural sea salt
2 teaspoons freshly ground black pepper
1 teaspoon cayenne pepper

The Protein Power of Egg Whites

Egg whites are the perfect blank canvas for the flavor and taste of additional ingredients—and they are one of the most protein-packed foods available. Egg whites also contain the essential vitamins and minerals that, when combined with other protein-rich foods, help the body's systems run efficiently for energy and recovery.

1. Preheat oven to 375°F.

2. Spray a 9" x 13" glass casserole dish with olive oil cooking spray.

3. Combine ground turkey breast, potatoes, egg whites, and eggs thoroughly.

4. Season with salt, black pepper, and cayenne.

5. Pour mixture into baking dish and let settle completely.

6. Bake for 30–40 minutes, or until top is golden and firm and inserted fork comes out clean.

PER SERVING Calories: 92 | Fat: 2.6 g | Protein: 11 g | Sodium: 387 mg | Fiber: 0.5 g | Carbohydrates: 6 g | Sugar: 0.2 g

Baked Apples and Cinnamon

Sweet apples and cinnamon combine for a wonderful, aromatic treat that is delicious served hot or cold. This healthy combination is the perfect sweet treat that's simple to make and a delectable indulgence.

INGREDIENTS | SERVES 6

6 apples, peeled, cored, and sliced
½ cup unsweetened applesauce
2 tablespoons agave nectar
2 teaspoons cinnamon

1. Preheat oven to 350°F.

2. Spray a 9" x 13" casserole dish with olive oil cooking spray.

3. Combine all ingredients in a mixing bowl, and stir to coat apples completely.

4. Cook for 30–40 minutes, or until apples are tender.

PER SERVING Calories: 96 | Fat: 0.3 g | Protein: 0 g | Sodium: 2 mg | Fiber: 3 g | Carbohydrates: 26 g | Sugar: 18 g

Cran-Orange Oatmeal

If your morning oatmeal has gotten a little boring, try this revamped version! Delicious cranberries and orange keep this classic treat healthy, but add zesty flavors that will make it anything but boring!

INGREDIENTS | SERVES 2

1 cup freshly squeezed orange juice (with pulp)
½ cup filtered water
1 cup cranberries
2 cups all-natural rolled oats
1 tablespoon freshly grated orange zest
1 tablespoon agave nectar

1. Combine orange juice, water, and cranberries in a medium saucepan over medium heat. Bring to a simmer.

2. Add oatmeal and simmer, stirring constantly, until it thickens, about 8 minutes.

3. Pour into two bowls, garnish with orange zest, and drizzle each with ½ tablespoon agave nectar.

PER SERVING Calories: 425 | Fat: 5.5 g | Protein: 12 g | Sodium: 11 mg | Fiber: 11 g | Carbohydrates: 85 g | Sugar: 22 g

Blazing Blueberry Muffins

Who doesn't love blueberry muffins?! Not only do these muffins smell and taste delicious, but the clean ingredients make them suitable for any diet or clean eater's delight.

INGREDIENTS | SERVES 12

¾ cup 100% whole wheat baking flour

¾ cup bran flakes cereal, crushed

½ cup Sucanat

½ teaspoon baking soda

1 teaspoon cinnamon

¼ cup unsweetened applesauce

1 cup mashed ripe bananas

½ cup vanilla almond milk

2 eggs

1 teaspoon vanilla extract

1 cup fresh blueberries

What Is Sucanat?

To adhere to the clean lifestyle, try to avoid refined sugars. Luckily, many unrefined, natural sweeteners are made from sugar cane juice. They're heated lightly and slowly to maintain nutrients, so your body can process them more efficiently than the white, refined alternative.

1. Preheat oven to 425°F.

2. Grease a 12-cup muffin pan or line with paper baking cups.

3. Combine flour, cereal, Sucanat, baking soda, and cinnamon in a large mixing bowl. Add applesauce, bananas, almond milk, eggs, and vanilla and mix well. Gently fold in blueberries.

4. Pour muffin mix evenly into each of the muffin cups.

5. Bake for 20 minutes, or until a fork inserted into the center of a muffin comes out clean.

PER SERVING Calories: 109 | Fat: 1.3 g | Protein: 3 g | Sodium: 35 mg | Fiber: 2.3 g | Carbohydrates: 23 g | Sugar: 12 g

Apple-Nana Muffins

Apples and bananas come together in these delicious muffins that will tantalize your taste buds and get any great day off to a great start!

INGREDIENTS | SERVES 12

¾ cup 100% whole wheat baking flour
¾ cup bran flakes cereal, crushed
½ cup Sucanat
½ teaspoon baking soda
1 teaspoon cinnamon
2 apples, peeled and cored
¼ cup unsweetened applesauce
1 cup mashed bananas
½ cup vanilla almond milk
2 eggs
1 teaspoon vanilla extract

Amazing Apples

Apples are wondrously versatile. Ranging from red to yellow to green, sweet to sour, and soft to crisp, you can tailor them to exactly what you want or need. Baking, sautéing, simmering, boiling, or leaving natural and raw, there's no bad way to prepare an apple!

1. Preheat oven to 375°F.

2. Slice apples and layer in a shallow baking dish. Add enough water to cover the bottom of the baking dish, and bake at 375°F for 20–30 minutes or until apples are fork-tender.

3. Grease a 12-cup muffin pan or line with paper baking cups.

4. Combine flour, cereal, Sucanat, baking soda, and cinnamon in a large mixing bowl. Add baked apples, applesauce, bananas, almond milk, eggs, and vanilla and mix well.

5. Pour muffin mix evenly into each of the muffin cups.

6. Bake for 20 minutes, or until a fork inserted into the center of a muffin comes out clean.

PER SERVING Calories: 113 | Fat: 14 g | Protein: 3 g | Sodium: 35 mg | Fiber: 2.5 g | Carbohydrates: 24 g | Sugar: 13 g

Cranberry Orange Bread

This colorful bread combines deliciously sweet and tart cranberries with the taste of orange.

INGREDIENTS | SERVES 12

1 cup 100% whole wheat baking flour

1 cup oat flour

½ cup Sucanat

1 teaspoon baking soda

½ teaspoon baking powder

1 cup mashed bananas

½ cup unsweetened applesauce

½ cup freshly squeezed orange juice

2 tablespoons freshly grated orange zest

4 egg whites

1 teaspoon vanilla

2 tablespoons agave nectar

1 cup cranberries

1. Preheat oven to 350°F.

2. Spray a loaf pan with olive oil spray and cover with a thin coating of wheat flour.

3. Combine flours, Sucanat, baking soda, and baking powder in a large mixing bowl.

4. Add bananas, applesauce, orange juice, zest, egg whites, vanilla, and agave nectar and mix well. Fold in cranberries.

5. Pour batter into the prepared pan and bake for 45–60 minutes, or until a knife inserted in the middle comes out clean.

PER SERVING Calories: 116 | Fat: 0.5 g | Protein: 3.7 g | Sodium: 46 mg | Fiber: 2.5 g | Carbohydrates: 26 g | Sugar: 15 g

Harness the Power of Cranberries

Cranberries contain lots of proanthrocy-anadins (naturally occurring compounds that can promote immunity, collagen production, and strength of the body's cellular structures). By preventing bacteria growth, cranberries might help prevent disorders such as urinary tract infections and ulcers.

Pumpkin Flaxseed Muffins

Contributing a lightly nutty background flavor, flaxseeds pair up with the bright taste of pumpkin in these hearty muffins that are delicious and health smart! They smell as heavenly as they taste.

INGREDIENTS | SERVES 12

¾ cup 100% whole wheat flour

½ cup ground flaxseed

½ cup Sucanat

½ teaspoon baking powder

1 teaspoon baking soda

1 teaspoon pumpkin pie spice

1½ cups pumpkin purée

½ cup vanilla almond milk

2 eggs

3 tablespoons agave nectar

1 teaspoon vanilla extract

Pumpkin for Optimum Health

This orange staple of fall festivals is packed with important antioxidants that promote health by building immunity. In addition, this winter squash is a great-tasting way to get a good dose of vitamin C.

1. Preheat oven to 375°F.

2. Grease a 12-cup muffin pan or line with paper baking cups.

3. Combine flour, flaxseed, Sucanat, baking powder, baking soda, and pumpkin pie spice in a large mixing bowl. Add pumpkin, almond milk, eggs, agave nectar, and vanilla. Blend well.

4. Pour muffin mix evenly into each of the muffin cups.

5. Bake for 20 minutes, or until a fork inserted into the center of a muffin comes out clean.

PER SERVING Calories: 138 | Fat: 4 g | Protein: 4 g | Sodium: 37 mg | Fiber: 3.3 g | Carbohydrates: 24 g | Sugar: 14 g

Sweet Potato Pancakes

You'll never look at pancakes the same way again once you taste this sweet potato variety! Sweet, smooth, and flavorful, this healthier option outdoes the refined favorite in every aspect.

INGREDIENTS | SERVES 10

1 cup sweet potato purée

1 cup plain low-fat Greek-style yogurt

1 cup unsweetened applesauce

2 egg whites

2 whole eggs

2 teaspoons vanilla

2 tablespoons Sucanat

¼ cup 100% whole wheat flour

1 teaspoon baking powder

1 teaspoon pumpkin pie spice

1 teaspoon cinnamon

2 tablespoons agave nectar

1. Coat a nonstick skillet with olive oil cooking spray and place over medium heat.

2. Combine all ingredients except agave nectar and mix well.

3. Scoop the batter onto the preheated skillet, using approximately ½ cup of batter per pancake.

4. Cook 2–3 minutes on each side, or until golden brown. Remove from heat, plate, and drizzle all pancakes with the agave nectar.

PER SERVING Calories: 78 | Fat: 1 g | Protein: 7 g | Sodium: 52 mg | Fiber: 1 g | Carbohydrates: 13 g | Sugar: 6 g

Almond Butter Sammies

Creamy almond butter and banana slices combine for delicious and healthy sandwiches that are a snap to make.

INGREDIENTS | SERVES 2

2 100% whole wheat English muffins, halved and toasted

4 tablespoons almond butter

1 banana, sliced

1. Spread each English muffin half with 1 tablespoon almond butter.

2. Top two muffin halves with banana slices.

3. Place other English muffin half on top and enjoy.

PER SERVING Calories: 316 | Fat: 9 g | Protein: 7.5 g | Sodium: 267 mg | Fiber: 4.5 g | Carbohydrates: 53 g | Sugar: 17 g

Banana Bread with Walnuts and Flaxseed

An age-old comfort food gets a makeover in this delicious recipe. This is a healthier version of the traditional treat—but it has the same great taste!

INGREDIENTS | SERVES 12

½ cup 100% whole wheat baking flour

½ cup oat flour

¾ cup ground flaxseed

½ cup Sucanat

1 teaspoon cinnamon

1 teaspoon baking soda

½ teaspoon baking powder

3 cups mashed bananas (about 3–4 medium-large bananas)

½ cup unsweetened applesauce

3 egg whites

1 whole egg

1 teaspoon vanilla extract

1 cup chopped natural walnuts

1. Preheat oven to 350°F.

2. Spray a loaf pan with olive oil cooking spray and cover with a thin coating of wheat flour.

3. In a large mixing bowl, combine flours, flaxseed, Sucanat, cinnamon, baking soda, and baking powder.

4. Add bananas, applesauce, egg whites, eggs, and vanilla. Mix to combine.

5. Incorporate walnuts evenly throughout the batter.

6. Pour batter into the prepared pan and bake for 45–60 minutes, or until a knife inserted in the middle comes out clean.

PER SERVING Calories: 215 | Fat: 10 g | Protein: 6.5 g | Sodium: 146 mg | Fiber: 5 g | Carbohydrates: 28 g | Sugar: 14 g

An Entire Day's Serving?!

Just ¼ cup of natural walnuts has almost an entire day's recommended value of omega 3s, an essential fatty acid our bodies can't produce that is critical for optimal brain and body system functioning! By gobbling up just a handful of these tasty treats, you are fueling your brain and your body.

Fruit-Stuffed French Toast Sandwiches

French toast can be loaded with fat and high in calories. This cleaned-up version uses healthier ingredients that not only deliver astounding health benefits, but make for one delicious version of a not-so-healthy favorite!

INGREDIENTS | SERVES 2

4 eggs, beaten

2 tablespoons vanilla almond milk

2 tablespoons agave nectar

4 slices sprouted grain bread

8 tablespoons sugar-free fruit spread

1 cup nonfat Greek-style yogurt

½ cup sliced strawberries

1 sliced banana

Sprouted Grain Bread

Sprouted grain breads are located in the frozen section of most grocery stores. They're a great option for the clean lifestyle because of their immense nutrition per slice—they contain about half the carb count of a slice of white bread. They use the sprouted germ of the wheat berry, thus the need for refrigeration.

1. Spray a large skillet with olive oil cooking spray and place over medium heat.

2. Whisk together the eggs, almond milk, and agave nectar.

3. Dip each bread slice in the egg mixture and place in heated skillet.

4. Cook each slice until lightly browned on each side and remove from heat.

5. Spread fruit spread evenly on one side of all bread slices, followed by a thin layer of yogurt. Layer the strawberries and bananas on two slices, and close the sandwiches by placing the other slices over the fruit.

6. Return the sandwiches to the heated frying pan and press down slightly.

7. Cook for 2–3 minutes and turn over. Continue cooking for 2–3 minutes or until both sides of the sandwiches are browned.

PER SERVING Calories: 452 | Fat: 12 g | Protein: 25 g | Sodium: 548 mg | Fiber: 3.4 g | Carbohydrates: 68 g | Sugar: 37 g

Garlicky Veggie-Packed Omelet

Delicious vegetables and garlic combine with fluffy eggs and egg whites to make a simple, satisfying, and savory meal that will start any day off right! Protein-packed and rich in complex carbohydrates from the vegetables, this is a tasty way to get some valuable nutrition.

INGREDIENTS | SERVES 1

¼ cup chopped onions
¼ cup mushrooms
2 tablespoons filtered water
2 teaspoons garlic powder
¼ cup torn spinach leaves
2 whole eggs
4 egg whites

Gracious Garlic

A member of the lily flower family, garlic is a beautiful plant that can give your meal a tantalizing aroma and a unique flavor. Use just a single clove of this versatile plant to dress up tasteless dishes, or create a savory flavor.

1. Coat a small frying pan with olive oil cooking spray and heat over medium heat.

2. Sauté onions for one minute. Add mushrooms and water, and continue sautéing until mushrooms are softened.

3. Sprinkle mixture with garlic powder and add the spinach leaves, stirring constantly.

4. Whisk together the eggs and egg whites and pour the egg mixture over the sautéed vegetables.

5. Immediately begin pulling the outer edges into the center for one turn around the whole pan. Let the omelet set for 2 minutes.

6. Slide the spatula under the omelet, gently lifting the center from the pan. Once the omelet is balancing on the spatula, quickly flip the omelet over.

7. Continue cooking the omelet for another 3–5 minutes, or until no juices remain when pressed upon.

PER SERVING Calories: 246 | Fat: 10 g | Protein: 29 g | Sodium: 371 mg | Fiber: 1.5 g | Carbohydrates: 10 g | Sugar: 4 g

Cinnamon Raisin Bread

Delicious cinnamon combines with all-natural raisins for a delicious treat with none of the guilt.

INGREDIENTS | SERVES 12

1 cup 100% whole wheat flour

½ cup ground flaxseeds

½ cup Sucanat

1 tablespoon cinnamon

1 teaspoon baking soda

½ teaspoon baking powder

2 cups mashed bananas (about 4 bananas)

¾ cup unsweetened applesauce

3 egg whites

1 egg

4 tablespoons agave nectar

1 teaspoon vanilla extract

1 cup raisins, natural and unsweetened

1 cup chopped natural walnuts

1. Preheat oven to 350°F. Spray a loaf pan with olive oil cooking spray and cover with a thin coating of wheat flour.

2. In a large mixing bowl, combine flour, flaxseeds, Sucanat, cinnamon, baking soda, and baking powder.

3. Add bananas, applesauce, egg whites, egg, agave nectar, and vanilla. Mix to combine. Fold in raisins and walnuts and incorporate evenly throughout the batter.

4. Pour batter into the prepared pan and bake for 45–60 minutes, or until a knife inserted in the middle comes out clean.

PER SERVING Calories: 218 | Fat: 8.6 g | Protein: 5 g | Sodium: 147 mg | Fiber: 4 g | Carbohydrates: 34 g | Sugar: 26 g

"Good" Carbohydrates

While there's still debate on whether "high-carb," "low-carb," or "no-carb" diets are beneficial, there's no debate on which carbs are best. Choose carbohydrates available in nature, such as fruits, vegetables, and whole grains, to ensure you get the most nutritional bang for your bite.

Sunshine Corn Muffins

These nutritious muffins get their sweetness from natural agave nectar rather than refined sugar.

INGREDIENTS | SERVES 12

1 cup 100% whole wheat flour

1 cup cornmeal

2 teaspoons baking soda

2 teaspoons baking powder

2 eggs

2 egg whites

½ cup unsweetened applesauce

3 tablespoons agave nectar

2 cups vanilla almond milk

½ cup plain nonfat yogurt

2 tablespoons canola oil

1 cup kernel corn (fresh or frozen)

Crunchy Cornmeal

Cornmeal can jazz up foods with a unique crunchy texture and taste. Try adding vegetables (raw or sautéed) to cornmeal breads and muffins, for a new way to eat your veggies! Low in fat, and a great source of energy, cornmeal is versatile, delicious, and nutritious.

1. Preheat oven to 425°F. Grease a 12-cup muffin pan or line with paper baking cups.

2. Combine flour, cornmeal, baking soda, and baking powder and mix thoroughly. Add eggs, egg whites, applesauce, agave nectar, almond milk, yogurt, and canola oil. Mix well.

3. Fold in the corn kernels, and spoon evenly into muffin cups.

4. Bake for 30–45 minutes, or until golden brown and inserted fork comes out clean.

PER SERVING Calories: 166 | Fat: 5 g | Protein: 5 g | Sodium: 386 mg | Fiber: 2.5 g | Carbohydrates: 26 g | Sugar: 6 g

Oat Bran Muffins

These deliciously dense muffins are hearty, tasty, and packed full of health benefits. Clean and filling is a great combination in this perfect breakfast on the go.

INGREDIENTS | SERVES 12

1 cup 100% whole wheat flour
½ cup crushed bran flakes
½ cup ground flaxseed
½ cup Sucanat
1 teaspoon baking soda
1 teaspoon baking powder
1½ teaspoons cinnamon
3 egg whites
1 egg
½ cup unsweetened applesauce
½ cup vanilla almond milk
1 tablespoon canola oil
3 tablespoons agave nectar
1 teaspoon vanilla
½ cup dry rolled oats

1. Preheat oven to 375°F. Grease a 12-cup muffin pan or line with paper baking cups.

2. Combine flour, bran flakes, flaxseed, Sucanat, baking soda, baking powder, and cinnamon in a large mixing bowl. Add egg whites, eggs, applesauce, almond milk, canola oil, agave nectar, and vanilla and mix well.

3. Pour muffin mix evenly into each of the muffin cups.

4. Sprinkle the ½ cup of oats over top, and press down lightly.

5. Bake for 20 minutes, or until a fork inserted into the center of a muffin comes out clean.

PER SERVING Calories: 114 | Fat: 3.8 g | Protein: 3 g | Sodium: 182 mg | Fiber: 2.5 g | Carbohydrates: 18 g | Sugar: 13 g

Bran 101

Many manufacturers of bran cereals now fortify their products with additional vitamins and minerals that aren't always easy to get in the standard American diet. Packed with iron and B vitamins, among many others, bran cereals can be a nutritious snack or healthy addition to baked good recipes.

Very Veggie Frittata

Packed with loads of protein from the egg whites and eggs, and rich in carbohydrates from all of the fresh vegetables, this is a great-tasting omelet. Customize it using your favorite veggies!

INGREDIENTS | SERVES 4

½ cup chopped broccoli
½ cup mushrooms, cleaned and diced
½ cup chopped yellow pepper
¼ onion, chopped finely
6 egg whites
6 eggs
1 tablespoon garlic powder
1 teaspoon all-natural sea salt
2 teaspoons freshly ground black pepper
¼ cup filtered water

1. Preheat oven to 350°F. Spray a large oven-safe skillet with olive oil cooking spray, and preheat over medium heat.

2. Combine broccoli, mushrooms, pepper, and onion in the skillet with the water and cook until tender, but not soft.

3. Whisk together egg whites, eggs, garlic powder, salt, and pepper and pour over veggie mixture.

4. Cook until the center begins to shake and bubble from the heat (about 3–4 minutes). Remove from heat and place in preheated oven for 15 minutes, or until center is set and an inserted fork comes out clean.

PER SERVING Calories: 181 | Fat: 8 g | Protein: 17 g | Sodium: 788 mg | Fiber: 4.5 g | Carbohydrates: 13 g | Sugar: 1.7 g

Heavenly Hash Browns

The classic high-fat version of this breakfast staple gets a complete overhaul in this delicious hash brown recipe. By using clean, fresh ingredients and replacing the not-so-wonderful oils with a small amount of olive oil, you can enjoy every last bite of these healthful hash browns.

INGREDIENTS | SERVES 6

3 medium Idaho potatoes, shredded

1 small yellow onion, minced

1 egg

2 tablespoons 100% whole wheat flour

1 teaspoon garlic powder

All-natural sea salt and freshly ground black pepper to taste

1 tablespoon olive oil

1. Spray a large skillet with olive oil cooking spray and preheat over medium heat.

2. In a large mixing bowl, combine shredded potatoes, onion, egg, flour, and garlic powder and mix until thoroughly blended. Add salt and pepper to taste.

3. Form potato mixture into dense patties, using ½ cup of the mixture for each patty.

4. Heat the olive oil in the skillet and add 2–3 hash brown patties at a time. Cook 3–5 minutes, or until golden brown.

5. Flip patties and continue cooking until golden brown on both sides and completely cooked through.

PER SERVING Calories: 130 | Fat: 3 g | Protein: 4 g | Sodium: 18 mg | Fiber: 2 g | Carbohydrates: 22.5 g | Sugar: 1.2 g

Jazzed Up Scramble Wrap Up

Perfect for a relaxing morning around the house, or as a breakfast to take with you in the car, these scrambled eggs are fragrant and full of flavor.

INGREDIENTS | SERVES 2

½ cup diced tomato

½ cup chopped spinach leaves

1 teaspoon garlic powder

1 teaspoon all-natural sea salt

1 teaspoon freshly ground black pepper

4 eggs

2 tablespoons filtered water

4 tablespoons nonfat plain yogurt

2 100% whole wheat tortillas

1. Coat a large skillet with olive oil cooking spray and preheat over medium heat.

2. Sauté the tomato and spinach leaves with the garlic powder, salt, and pepper until spinach is wilted.

3. In a small mixing bowl, beat eggs and water. Pour eggs over vegetables and scramble until light and fluffy in consistency.

4. Spread 2 tablespoons of the yogurt down the center of each tortilla and top with the egg and vegetable mixture.

5. Wrap tightly and enjoy!

PER SERVING Calories: 272 | Fat: 13 g | Protein: 17 g | Sodium: 978 mg | Fiber: 2 g | Carbohydrates: 21 g | Sugar: 4 g

Protein-Packed Breakfast Burritos

These burritos are great for breakfast or as a protein power up following an intense workout.

INGREDIENTS | SERVES 2

½ red pepper, diced

1 small jalapeño, seeds removed, and sliced or chopped

½ yellow onion, diced

4 eggs

2 tablespoons filtered water

2 100% whole wheat tortillas

1 cup Spicy Clean Refried Beans (see recipe in Chapter 4)

2 tablespoons Greek-style nonfat yogurt

¼ cup shredded romaine lettuce

¼ cup diced tomatoes

1. Coat a large skillet with olive oil spray and preheat over medium heat.

2. Sauté red pepper, jalapeño, and onions until cooked, but not soft.

3. Beat together eggs and water and pour over the vegetables. Scramble together until light and fluffy.

4. Lay out two tortillas and spread ½ cup of the spicy refried beans on each.

5. Top beans with 1 tablespoon of the yogurt and layer eggs on top.

6. Sprinkle lettuce and tomato on top of each and wrap tightly.

PER SERVING Calories: 375 | Fat: 14 g | Protein: 23 g | Sodium: 877 mg | Fiber: 8.6 g | Carbohydrates: 41 g | Sugar: 5.4 g

Fruity Yogurt Parfaits

Super simple and delicious, these parfaits are a light breakfast
option that leaves no nutritional element out.

INGREDIENTS | SERVES 2

2 cups plain low-fat yogurt

1 cup "Good Gracious!" Granola (see recipe in Chapter 4)

2 sliced bananas

½ cup blueberries

½ cup sliced strawberries

Yogurt for All

Whatever your taste and consistency preferences, there's a yogurt out there that you'll like. This protein-packed, probiotic snack helps promote a healthy metabolism, fuels the body and mind, and builds up protection against harmful bacteria growth. What more could you ask for?

1. Place ⅓ cup of yogurt in the bottom of two 16-ounce glasses.

2. Top each with ¼ cup granola, ½ sliced banana, and ¼ cup blueberries.

3. Layer another ⅓ cup of yogurt, followed by ¼ cup granola, ½ sliced banana, and ¼ cup strawberries.

4. Top with remaining yogurt.

PER SERVING Calories: 397 | Fat: 2.5 g | Protein: 19 g | Sodium: 307 mg | Fiber: 6.8 g | Carbohydrates: 80 g | Sugar: 50 g

CHAPTER 3

Smoothies

Strawberry Dream

Clean carbohydrates and protein are packed into this smoothie. The simplicity and sweetness of carbs is sure to make this smoothie a delicious treat for kids and adults alike!

INGREDIENTS | SERVES 2

2 cups strawberries

1 cup strawberry kefir

1 teaspoon vanilla extract

1 cup ice

1. Combine strawberries, kefir, and vanilla extract in the blender with ½ cup of the ice, and blend until thoroughly combined.

2. Add remaining ice slowly while blending until desired consistency is reached.

PER SERVING Calories: 127 | Fat: 4 g | Protein: 5 g | Sodium: 60 mg | Fiber: 4 g | Carbohydrates: 18 g | Sugar: 13 g

Creamy Kefir's Amazing Nutrition

Kefir is a delightful blend of fruit, dairy, and plentiful probiotics. It contains more protein than milk, plus "good" bacteria, low fat and calorie counts, and enzymes that optimize your body's functioning. Try plain, strawberry, cherry, and vanilla!

Berry Banana

Whether a breakfast treat or an afternoon pick-me-up, this amazing smoothie is sure to be a sensation for the senses.

INGREDIENTS | SERVES 2

2 bananas, peeled

1 cup strawberries

1 cup blueberries

1 cup strawberry kefir

1 teaspoon vanilla extract

2 cups ice

1. Combine bananas, berries, kefir, and vanilla extract in the blender with 1 cup of the ice and blend until thoroughly combined.

2. Add remaining cup of ice gradually while blending until desired consistency is reached.

PER SERVING Calories: 252 | Fat: 4.5 g | Protein: 6 g | Sodium: 61 mg | Fiber: 7.5 g | Carbohydrates: 50 g | Sugar: 31 g

Packed with Potassium

Bananas do much more than just taste great. They're full of potassium, a mineral that most people don't get enough of. Potassium can promote cardiovascular health by preventing high blood pressure!

Very Cherry Vanilla

If you never thought your kids would go for natural cherries (not the processed maraschino kind!), you may be surprised at their delight with this confectionary concoction.

INGREDIENTS | SERVES 2

2 cups cherries, pitted

1 banana, peeled

Pulp of 1 vanilla bean

1 cup of vanilla almond milk

1 teaspoon vanilla extract

1 cup of ice

1. Combine cherries, bananas, vanilla bean pulp, almond milk, and vanilla extract in the blender with ½ cup of the ice and blend until thoroughly combined.

2. Add remaining ½ cup of ice gradually while blending until desired consistency is reached.

PER SERVING Calories: 200 | Fat: 4.5 g | Protein: 3.5 g | Sodium: 202 mg | Fiber: 6 g | Carbohydrates: 40 g | Sugar: 27 g

Where to Find Vanilla Beans

Vanilla beans can be found at your local grocery store, with other dried herbs and/ or baking essentials. Slit the bean down the center with a sharp knife, open the skin, and reveal the pulp; this pulp is the ingredient referred to in most cookbooks.

Pumpkin Spice

If you're looking for an escape from the usual fruit smoothie, mix things up with this delicious pumpkin pie in a glass! Raw ingredients and aromatic spices make this clean smoothie the most delicious and healthy dessert option around.

INGREDIENTS | SERVES 2

1 cup sweet potato purée

1 cup vanilla almond milk

1 teaspoon ground cloves

1 teaspoon ginger

1 teaspoon cinnamon

2 cups of ice

1. Combine sweet potato, almond milk, and spices in the blender with 1 cup of the ice and blend until thoroughly combined.

2. Add remaining cup of ice gradually while blending until desired consistency is reached.

PER SERVING Calories: 118 | Fat: 4 g | Protein: 2.5 g | Sodium: 227 mg | Fiber: 3.8 g | Carbohydrates: 19 g | Sugar: 4.6 g

Mango Madness

Since mangoes are now available frozen year-round, try this treat any time of year.

INGREDIENTS | SERVES 2

1 cup chopped mango
1 large banana, peeled
1 cup vanilla almond milk
2 cups ice

Mangoes Year-Round

If you can't find mangoes fresh out of season, look in your grocer's freezer. This vibrant fruit can be enjoyed year-round thanks to the manufacturers who have prepared, peeled, flash-frozen, and packaged this delicious treat into handy organic packages.

1. Combine mango, banana, and almond milk in the blender with ½ cup of the ice and blend until thoroughly combined.

2. Add remaining ice gradually while blending until desired consistency is reached.

PER SERVING Calories: 158 | Fat: 4 g | Protein: 2.2 g | Sodium: 203 mg | Fiber: 4.5 g | Carbohydrates: 31 g | Sugar: 20 g

Peaches 'n Cream

All clean, all healthy, and all absolutely delicious, these ingredients make for a fabulous treat.

INGREDIENTS | SERVES 2

2 cups fresh chopped peaches
1 banana, peeled
2 cups vanilla almond milk
2 cups ice

1. Combine peaches, banana, and almond milk in the blender with ½ cup of the ice and blend until thoroughly combined.

2. Add remaining ice gradually while blending until desired consistency is reached.

PER SERVING Calories: 202 | Fat: 8.4 g | Protein: 4.2 g | Sodium: 403 mg | Fiber: 6 g | Carbohydrates: 32 g | Sugar: 20 g

Pineapple Delight

Perky pineapple can bring anyone's senses to attention. Some kids steer clear of whole pineapple, but you may be pleasantly surprised when your whole family loves the taste of this pineapple and coconut milk blend.

INGREDIENTS | SERVES 2

2 cups fresh pineapple (about one large)

2 cups coconut milk (such as Silk Pure Coconut Milk)

2 cups ice

1. Combine pineapple and coconut milk in the blender with ½ cup of the ice and blend until thoroughly combined.

2. Add remaining ice gradually while blending until desired consistency is reached.

PER SERVING Calories: 157 | Fat: 5 g | Protein: 2 g | Sodium: 31 mg | Fiber: 2 g | Carbohydrates: 28 g | Sugar: 16 g

Pineapple for Promoting Health

Topping the charts for its exceptional doses of manganese, vitamin C, and B vitamins, pineapple is worth its weight in health benefits. Indulging in this delicious fruit provides protection against illness and promotes top brain functioning and quick metabolism.

All Almonds

Going nutty with this smoothie is perfectly fine! Almonds and aromatic vanilla become even more delicious with the scrumptious addition of bananas and nutmeg.

INGREDIENTS | SERVES 2

2 cups whole, unsalted almonds

2 cups filtered water

2 bananas, peeled

Pulp of 1 vanilla bean

1 teaspoon nutmeg

2 cups ice

1. Emulsify the almonds and water until no bits of the almond remain, and the mixture is thoroughly combined.

2. Add the bananas, vanilla bean pulp, and nutmeg in the blender with ½ cup of the ice and blend until thoroughly combined.

3. Add remaining ice gradually while blending until desired consistency is reached.

PER SERVING Calories: 657 | Fat: 47 g | Protein: 21 g | Sodium: 9.4 mg | Fiber: 15 g | Carbohydrates: 48 g | Sugar: 18 g

Homemade Almond Milk

If you reach for the almond milk and realize you're out, don't despair. All you need is 2 cups of natural, unsalted almonds; 2 cups of filtered water; and a powerful blender. Simply blend the combination until no bits remain. Ta-da!

Chocolate Almond Butter

Chocolate lovers rejoice! Any sweet tooth's cravings can be satisfied with this healthy—but still sinfully chocolaty—smoothie. Delicious and nutritious, this smoothie appeals to all lovers of the smooth chocolate and peanut butter combination . . . especially kids!

INGREDIENTS | SERVES 2

1 banana, peeled
4 dates, pitted
¼ cup raw cocoa
½ cup natural almond butter
2 cups vanilla almond milk
2 cups ice

1. Combine the banana, dates, cocoa, almond butter, and almond milk in the blender with ½ cup of the ice and blend until thoroughly combined.

2. Add remaining ice gradually while blending until desired consistency is reached.

PER SERVING Calories: 473 | Fat: 25 g | Protein: 10.5 g | Sodium: 411 mg | Fiber: 11 g | Carbohydrates: 63 g | Sugar: 38 g

The Rundown on Raw Cocoa

Packed with powerful antioxidants, raw cocoa is a nutritious alternative to sugar-laden and calorie-clouded milk chocolate. Blending the raw cocoa in a smoothie that contains flavorful ingredients will sweeten up the cocoa without masking it.

Tropical Paradise

This smoothie is worthy of those cute little drink umbrellas. The combination of tropical fruit makes for a light and satisfying smoothie that will rejuvenate your energy and awaken your taste buds!

INGREDIENTS | SERVES 2

1½ cups coconut meat, mashed and softened
1 cup fresh pineapple
½ cup mango
1 clementine, peeled
2 cups coconut milk
2 cups ice

1. Combine coconut, pineapple, mango, clementine, and coconut milk in the blender with ½ cup of the ice and blend until thoroughly combined.

2. Add remaining ice gradually while blending until desired consistency is reached.

PER SERVING Calories: 754 | Fat: 68 g | Protein: 7.6 g | Sodium: 44 mg | Fiber: 8 g | Carbohydrates: 40 g | Sugar: 24 g

Clean Green Go-Getter

While getting enough fiber can be a daunting task, this smoothie recipe makes it easy. Fibrous veggies make for an easy-to-drink—and easy-to-digest—one-stop meal option.

INGREDIENTS | SERVES 2

1 cup spinach
½ cup broccoli florets
½ cup cauliflower florets
2 garlic cloves
2 cups filtered water
2 cups ice

1. Combine spinach, broccoli, cauliflower, garlic, and 1½ cups of water in the blender with 1 cup of the ice and blend until thoroughly combined.

2. Add remaining water and ice gradually while blending until desired consistency is reached.

PER SERVING Calories: 21 | Fat: 0.2 g | Protein: 1.7 g | Sodium: 34 mg | Fiber: 1.5 g | Carbohydrates: 4.2 g | Sugar: 1 g

Crazy Coconut

When was the last time you enjoyed a coconut creation without the alcohol? This clean recipe gives you all the taste with none of the hangover!

INGREDIENTS | SERVES 2

2 cups processed coconut meat (sold in cans)
1 banana, peeled
1 cup coconut milk
2 cups ice

1. Combine processed coconut meat, banana, and coconut milk in the blender with ½ cup of the ice and blend until thoroughly combined.

2. Add remaining ice gradually while blending until desired consistency is reached.

PER SERVING Calories: 558 | Fat: 51 g | Protein: 6 g | Sodium: 31 mg | Fiber: 9 g | Carbohydrates: 29 g | Sugar: 12 g

Oatmeal Berry

Hearty oatmeal combines with sweet berries and flavorful blueberry kefir for one amazing smoothie combination that can be the perfect breakfast or dessert.

INGREDIENTS | SERVES 2

1 cup blueberries

1 cup raspberries

½ cup dry rolled oats

2½ cups blueberry kefir

2 teaspoons cinnamon

2 cups ice

1. Combine berries, oats, kefir, and cinnamon in the blender with ½ cup of the ice and blend until thoroughly combined.

2. Add remaining ice gradually while blending until desired consistency is reached.

PER SERVING Calories: 345 | Fat: 11 g | Protein: 13 g | Sodium: 148 mg | Fiber: 12.5 g | Carbohydrates: 51 g | Sugar: 24 g

Creamy Blueberry

Blueberry muffins, make way for the new kid in town! No need for the baking time or cleanup with this one-stop smoothie that packs a punch with flavor and amazing health benefits.

INGREDIENTS | SERVES 2

2 cups blueberries

2 bananas, peeled

½ cup vanilla almond milk

1½ cups blueberry kefir

1 teaspoon vanilla extract

2 cups ice

1. Combine blueberries, bananas, almond milk, kefir, and vanilla extract in the blender with ½ cup of the ice and blend until thoroughly combined.

2. Add remaining ice gradually while blending until desired consistency is reached.

PER SERVING Calories: 331 | Fat: 8.4 g | Protein: 8.5 g | Sodium: 191 mg | Fiber: 9.2 g | Carbohydrates: 60 g | Sugar: 37 g

Have You Had Your Anthocyanins Today?

Found in blueberries, phytochemicals such as anthocyanins are fierce warriors in the battle against free radicals and protect your body from damage to your eyes, skin, brain, and immune system.

Perfect Pear

Pears rarely get the attention they deserve. This smoothie will remind you of why you loved pears . . . and make you wonder why you haven't been enjoying them as much until now.

INGREDIENTS | SERVES 2

3 pears, peeled and cored

1 banana, peeled

1 cup vanilla almond milk

1 teaspoon cinnamon

2 cups ice

Pears for Fiber

Aside from the abundant vitamins and minerals like vitamins B and C, folic acid, niacin, phosphorus, and calcium, pears are a great source of fiber. A clean diet with adequate fiber will ensure that any gastrointestinal issues are a thing of the past.

1. Slice the pears and layer in a shallow baking dish. Add enough water to cover the bottom of the baking dish, and bake at 375°F for 20–30 minutes or until pears are fork-tender.

2. Combine cooked pears, banana, almond milk, and cinnamon in the blender with ½ cup of the ice and blend until thoroughly combined.

3. Add remaining ice gradually while blending until desired consistency is reached.

PER SERVING Calories: 244 | Fat: 4.5 g | Protein: 3 g | Sodium: 204 mg | Fiber: 11 g | Carbohydrates: 55 g | Sugar: 32 g

Savory Spinach and Garlic

You may not think of spinach and garlic as typical smoothie ingredients, but it's time to think outside the box! Give this smoothie a try as a light afternoon snack.

INGREDIENTS | SERVES 2

1 cup spinach leaves

2 tomatoes, chopped

3 cloves garlic

2 cups filtered water

2 cups ice

Spinach for Vitamins and Minerals

Get your daily recommended number of veggies with spinach, which is packed with folate and iron. A salad here, a spinach-stuffed dinner there, and an occasional spinach smoothie can help you check off your vegetable servings simply and deliciously.

1. Combine spinach, tomatoes, garlic, and water in the blender with ½ cup of the ice and blend until thoroughly combined.

2. Add remaining ice gradually while blending until desired consistency is reached.

PER SERVING Calories: 32 | Fat: 0.3 g | Protein: 1.8 g | Sodium: 26 mg | Fiber: 2 g | Carbohydrates: 7 g | Sugar: 3.4 g

Apple Pie

Smooth, satisfying, aromatic, and absolutely mouthwatering, this smoothie packs all the healthiest ingredients into a tasty treat that will calm your craving for the calorie- and fat-laden version of apple pie! It's not only a great guilt-free treat for you, but for kids, too!

INGREDIENTS | SERVES 2

3 apples, cored
1 banana, peeled
1 teaspoon cinnamon
1 teaspoon cloves
1 teaspoon nutmeg
1 teaspoon ginger
1 teaspoon vanilla
2 cups vanilla almond milk
2 cups ice

1. Slice apples and layer in a shallow baking dish. Add water to cover the bottom of the baking dish, and bake at 375°F for 20–30 minutes or until apples are fork-tender.

2. Combine cooked apples, banana, cinnamon, cloves, nutmeg, ginger, vanilla, and almond milk in the blender with ½ cup of the ice and blend until thoroughly combined.

3. Add remaining ice gradually while blending until desired consistency is reached.

PER SERVING Calories: 279 | Fat: 9 g | Protein: 3.8 g | Sodium: 407 mg | Fiber: 8 g | Carbohydrates: 52 g | Sugar: 32 g

Chocolate Peanut Butter Delight

Getting its chocolaty taste from emulsified dates, this smoothie takes a calorie-packed, fat-laden diet trap and transforms it into a delicious healthy treat. Morning (I won't tell!), noon, or night, this smoothie will calm those chocolate–peanut butter cravings!

INGREDIENTS | SERVES 2

5 dates, pitted
4 tablespoons almond butter
2 cups vanilla almond milk
2 cups ice

1. Combine the dates, 1 cup of almond milk, and ½ of the ice in a blender, and blend until the dates are emulsified.

2. Add the almond butter, remaining cup of almond milk, and remaining ice while blending until desired consistency is achieved.

PER SERVING Calories: 278 | Fat: 15.8 g | Protein: 5.3 g | Sodium: 406 mg | Fiber: 5 g | Carbohydrates: 34 g | Sugar: 23 g

Dates Instead of Chocolate

Although you may find it surprising, dates (the dried version of figs) can be used in many recipes as a substitute for chocolate. Lending a delicious sweetness and smoothness that's amazingly similar to chocolate, dates offer up more nutrition, important daily fruit servings, and no sugar crash!

Cherry Banana Protein Power

The unique combination of cherry and banana is more than tasty—it's good for you! This smoothie packs tons of protein and zero guilt.

INGREDIENTS | SERVES 2

1 large banana, peeled

1 cup cherries, pitted

2 cups vanilla almond milk

1 cup ice

1. Combine banana, cherries, and almond milk in a blender with ½ cup of ice and blend until thoroughly combined.

2. Add remaining ½ cup of ice as needed while blending until desired consistency is achieved.

PER SERVING Calories: 198 | Fat: 8 g | Protein: 3.7 g | Sodium: 403 mg | Fiber: 5.6 g | Carbohydrates: 32 g | Sugar: 18 g

Sour Apple

Tart lemons and sweet apples combine in this delicious "wake-me-up" smoothie that will liven up any sluggish morning or slow-moving day. This one will grab your attention for its unique flavors.

INGREDIENTS | SERVES 2

2 Granny Smith apples, peeled and cored

1 lemon, peeled and seeds removed

1 cup filtered water

2 tablespoons agave nectar

1 cup ice

1. Combine apples, lemon, and water in the blender container and blend until thoroughly combined with no apple bits remaining.

2. Add ice while blending until desired consistency is achieved.

3. Drizzle in 1 tablespoon agave and blend. Taste and add remaining agave until desired sweetness is achieved.

PER SERVING Calories: 116 | Fat: 0.2 g | Protein: 0.6 g | Sodium: 6 mg | Fiber: 2.8 g | Carbohydrates: 32 g | Sugar: 27 g

Lime Chiller

Containing an amazingly low amount of calories, this tasty treat is a guiltless pleasure.

INGREDIENTS | SERVES 2

2 limes, peeled and seeds removed

1 tablespoon agave nectar

1 cup filtered water

1 cup ice

1. Combine limes, agave, water, and ½ cup of the ice in a blender and blend until thoroughly combined.

2. Add remaining ½ cup of ice while blending until desired consistency is achieved.

PER SERVING Calories: 52 | Fat: 0.1 g | Protein: 0.5 g | Sodium: 1.7 mg | Fiber: 2 g | Carbohydrates: 16 g | Sugar: 9.8 g

Mega Melon

The cool and lightly sweet refreshment that can only come from fresh melons is bursting out of this smoothie. This smoothie is the perfect treat on any hot afternoon . . . for adults and kids, too!

INGREDIENTS | SERVES 2

½ cantaloupe, rind and seeds removed

½ honeydew melon, rind and seeds removed

½ cup filtered water

1½ cups ice

1. Combine cantaloupe, honeydew, water, and ½ of the ice in a blender, and blend until thoroughly combined.

2. Add remaining ice while blending until desired consistency is achieved.

PER SERVING Calories: 136 | Fat: 0.6 g | Protein: 2.5 g | Sodium: 67 mg | Fiber: 3.2 g | Carbohydrates: 34 g | Sugar: 31 g

Hydrating Melons

Fruit smoothies are a tasty way to hydrate, and including melons in your delicious snack makes them that much more thirst-quenching. Packed with amazing amounts of vitamins and nutrients, these healthy fruits add tons of hydrating juices to any blended drink!

Lots of Latte

Using real coffee in this delicious smoothie allows you to include your traditional morning cup of joe in a clean way. Combining the antioxidant-rich coffee with protein-packed almond milk makes this a healthier version of the cream-laden cup you've become accustomed to.

INGREDIENTS | SERVES 2

2 cups prepared coffee, cooled

2 cups vanilla almond milk

2–3 cups ice

1 tablespoon agave nectar

Caffeinated Antioxidants

Coffee lovers rejoice—many scientists have deemed your morning pick-me-up a good thing. It's packed with antioxidants that promote health and protect against dangerous free radical damage. So whip up a smoothie that combines the delicious brew with clean ingredients.

1. Combine the coffee, almond milk, and ½ of the ice in a blender, and blend until thoroughly combined.

2. Add remaining ice while blending until desired consistency is achieved.

3. Add agave nectar gradually while blending until desired sweetness is achieved.

PER SERVING Calories: 124 | Fat: 7.8 g | Protein: 2.5 g | Sodium: 408 mg | Fiber: 2.3 g | Carbohydrates: 13 g | Sugar: 8.7 g

CHAPTER 4

Snacks

Buffalo Drumsticks

Buffalo wings can be an unexpected fat trap. Rather than fried and dressed in fat- and sodium-laden sauces, these spicy drumsticks provide healthy helpings of clean protein and delicious taste without any of the downfalls of the restaurant variety.

INGREDIENTS | SERVES 12

12 skinless organic chicken drumsticks

1 cup unsweetened almond milk

3 tablespoons cayenne pepper

Cayenne for Hot and Spicy Flavor

Storebought versions of hot sauce, and even some homemade versions, can contain loads of sodium and sugar. By using spices like cayenne pepper, you can achieve a hot and spicy kick to any dish without any additives that may be detrimental to your health.

1. Place drumsticks in a gallon-sized resealable plastic bag with the almond milk and marinate for 1–2 hours.

2. Discard almond milk from bag, and pour 2 tablespoons of the cayenne pepper into the bag and reseal.

3. Toss the drumsticks to coat evenly.

4. Preheat oven to 400°F, and place drumsticks onto foil-lined baking sheet prepared with olive oil spray.

5. Sprinkle remaining tablespoon of cayenne onto drumsticks.

6. Cook for 20–25 minutes or until crispy.

PER SERVING Calories: 132 | Fat: 7 g | Protein: 15 g | Sodium: 71 mg | Fiber: 0.5 g | Carbohydrates: 2 g | Sugar: 1 g

Coconut Chicken Fingers

Anything but ordinary, these delicious chicken fingers are marinated in pineapple and coconut milk, and dressed in scrumptious crunchy coconut flakes for a taste that's sure to impress. These juicy and flavorful tenders are sweet enough to be a hit with kids, too!

INGREDIENTS | SERVES 12

12 organic chicken tenders

½ cup coconut milk

½ cup fresh pineapple juice

2 cups all-natural, unsweetened coconut flakes

Coconut Flakes

If you're looking for a healthy sprinkling of deliciousness to add to a favorite meal, reach no further than to a heaping helping of natural coconut flakes. Unsweetened varieties of coconut flakes are packed with tons of flavor without the added sugar. Toasted at home for added crunchiness, you can use these delicious flakes as a topping or a great addition to cookies or even as a delicious sweet contrast to savory entrées.

1. Place tenders in a gallon resealable plastic bag with coconut milk and pineapple juice, and marinate for 1–2 hours.

2. Preheat oven to 400°F. Pour coconut flakes into a shallow dish.

3. Move the tenders from the marinade bag to the coconut flake dish and coat them evenly.

4. Arrange the tenders onto a foil-lined baking sheet prepared with olive oil spray.

5. Cook for 20–25 minutes or until crispy.

PER SERVING Calories: 296 | Fat: 27 g | Protein: 15 g | Sodium: 80 mg | Fiber: 6 g | Carbohydrates: 10 g | Sugar: 4 g

Quickie Quesadillas

The quesadilla loses its nutritional appeal if you pack in creams and cheeses and leave out vegetables. This revved-up wonder includes chicken and veggies, protein-packed yogurt, and delicious spices all wrapped in whole wheat tortillas for a snack that gives back!

INGREDIENTS | SERVES 2

2 100% whole wheat tortillas

4 tablespoons plain Greek-style yogurt

1 teaspoon freshly ground black pepper

1 teaspoon garlic powder

1 teaspoon onion powder

1 teaspoon all-natural sea salt

1 cup cooked chicken, torn

1 cup steamed broccoli, in bite-sized pieces

1. Lay tortillas on a flat surface, and spread 2 tablespoons of the Greek yogurt over each one evenly. Sprinkle half of each of the spices on each tortilla.

2. Layer the chicken and broccoli evenly on one half of each tortilla and fold in half over toppings.

3. Toast in a toaster oven for 4 minutes on each side, or broil at 450°F for 2 minutes on each side, watching constantly.

PER SERVING Calories: 264 | Fat: 7.7 g | Protein: 25 g | Sodium: 1263 mg | Fiber: 2.6 g | Carbohydrates: 23 g | Sugar: 3.5 g

Roasted Red Pepper Hummus

This tasty combination of roasted red peppers and hearty chickpeas will satisfy any hunger pains! This snack pairs great with Tasty Tortilla Chips (see recipe in this chapter) for an energy-boosting snack!

INGREDIENTS | SERVES 12

1 cup chickpeas, soaked for 12 hours

1 roasted red pepper

2 cloves garlic

1 cup olive oil

¼ cup freshly squeezed lime juice

1 teaspoon all-natural sea salt

1 teaspoon cayenne pepper

1 cup filtered water

1. Combine chickpeas, roasted red pepper, garlic cloves, olive oil, lime juice, salt, and cayenne pepper in a blender or food processor.

2. Emulsify ingredients into a thick paste.

3. Add water gradually until desired consistency is achieved.

PER SERVING Calories: 207 | Fat: 18 g | Protein: 2.5 g | Sodium: 200 mg | Fiber: 2.3 g | Carbohydrates: 8 g | Sugar: 1.4 g

Fruit Salad Pizza

Sometimes you just can't ignore a sweet tooth. Whether you're not satisfied with a delicious smoothie, or just having a hankering for some sweet carbs, this snack will do the trick. An all-natural crust, creamy yogurt, and fresh fruit gather together for one unique snack.

INGREDIENTS | SERVES 8

4 cups natural pecans

⅓ cup dates

⅔ cup coconut oil

1 cup vanilla nonfat Greek-style yogurt

⅓ cup freshly squeezed orange juice

4 tablespoons agave nectar

1 cup sliced strawberries

2 kiwis, sliced thinly

2 clementine oranges, peeled and separated

½ cup chopped pineapple

1 cup fresh blueberries

The Fuzzy Forgotten Fruit

Because of their very different flavor and texture, kiwis aren't always included in fruity blends. Making for a very delicious addition to any kind of salad, smoothie, or main entrée, kiwis have vitamins A and C, as well as potassium.

1. Combine the pecans, dates, and coconut oil in a food processor. Process until smooth, and form into a crust in a 9" x 13" glass dish.

2. Mix together the yogurt, orange juice, and 2 tablespoons of the agave nectar. Layer the mixture on top of the nut crust.

3. Assemble the fruit with the sliced strawberries on the outer edge of the entire pan, followed by the kiwis and clementines in separate rows moving inward.

4. Scatter the pineapple and blueberries to fill the center, and top by drizzling the remaining 2 tablespoons of agave.

PER SERVING Calories: 640 | Fat: 57 g | Protein: 7 g | Sodium: 18 mg | Fiber: 7.4 g | Carbohydrates: 33 g | Sugar: 22 g

Honey Mustard Chicken Tenders

Some honey mustard recipes can be laden with sugar and sodium, but this recipe ditches the bad stuff while keeping the great taste. Sweet and tangy, these tenders are great as a snack or cut up for sharing as an appetizer.

INGREDIENTS | SERVES 6

12 organic chicken tenders

5 tablespoons agave nectar

2 tablespoons plus 1 teaspoon dry mustard

1 teaspoon all-natural sea salt

Homemade Honey Mustard

To make your own honey mustard, combine fresh agave nectar and ground dry mustard, then tweak the amounts until you achieve the flavor you want. The best part: no poor ingredients, no added sodium or preservatives, and only two ingredients that you don't have difficulty pronouncing.

1. In a large resealable plastic bag, combine chicken tenders, 4 tablespoons of the agave, and 2 tablespoons of the dry mustard. Toss to coat and marinate 1 hour.

2. Prepare a baking sheet with aluminum foil and olive oil spray and preheat oven to 400°F.

3. Line chicken tenders on prepared baking sheet. Drizzle remaining tablespoon of agave and teaspoon of dry mustard over tenders.

4. Bake for 20 minutes, or until tenders are golden brown.

PER SERVING Calories: 185 | Fat: 3 g | Protein: 24 g | Sodium: 592 mg | Fiber: 0.2 g | Carbohydrates: 15 g | Sugar: 14 g

Tasty Tortilla Chips

Rather than opting for the bagged variety, make your own tortilla chips! Customize them to your liking with fresh ingredients and flavorful herbs and spices. Save money, a trip to the grocery store, and all those added sodium and preservatives!

INGREDIENTS | SERVES 32

8 100% whole wheat tortillas

2 tablespoons olive oil

1 tablespoon each salt, pepper, and/or seasoning (of choice)

1. Preheat oven to 350°F and prepare a baking sheet with foil and olive oil spray.

2. Cut each tortilla into 8 pizza-shaped slices.

3. Arrange the tortillas evenly on the baking sheet.

4. Lightly drizzle the chips with olive oil and sprinkle with desired seasoning, or just salt and pepper.

5. Bake for 8–10 minutes, or until crispy.

PER SERVING Calories: 31 | Fat: 1.5 g | Protein: 0.6 g | Sodium: 268 mg | Fiber: 0.3 g | Carbohydrates: 3.8 g | Sugar: 0.1 g

Fish Fingers

Thankfully, you can leave the processed and unidentifiable fish sticks of your childhood where they belong . . . in the past. Fresh fish makes a star appearance worthy of greatness in these delicious sticks that are quick, easy, and absolutely amazing!

INGREDIENTS | SERVES 10

1 pound tilapia or cod fillets

½ cup freshly squeezed lime juice

2 tablespoons 100% whole wheat flour

1 teaspoon all-natural sea salt

1 teaspoon freshly ground black pepper

1 teaspoon garlic powder

Fresh vs. Storebought Fish Sticks

Although manufacturers have made it easy on parents by providing frozen fish sticks that can be ready on a moment's notice, you should still consider their ingredients and preparation methods. Figure out the type of fish used and how it was raised, the ingredients in the breading, and the preparation methods from start to finish. Making fresh fish sticks yourself is the healthiest way to serve up these omega-rich treats to your little ones . . . without concern or guilt.

1. Cut fillets into 10 1"-thick pieces and place into a large resealable plastic bag with lime juice. Refrigerate and marinate for 30 minutes.

2. Preheat oven to 400°F, and prepare a baking sheet with aluminum foil and olive oil spray. Place flour in a shallow dish, and dredge fish sticks to coat evenly.

3. Line dredged fish fingers on the baking sheet and sprinkle with the salt, pepper, and garlic powder.

4. Bake for 20 minutes, or until crust is golden brown and fish is flaky.

PER SERVING Calories: 47 | Fat: 0.4 g | Protein: 8 g | Sodium: 260 mg | Fiber: 0.5 g | Carbohydrates: 2.6 g | Sugar: 0.2 g

Burger Bites

Ground turkey breast, seasoned perfectly and grilled just right, pairs up with all the fixin's for a great satisfying snack that will calm any craving for a greasy alternative.

INGREDIENTS | SERVES 8

1 yellow onion, diced

1 tablespoon minced garlic

2 tablespoons filtered water

1 pound ground turkey breast

1 teaspoon all-natural sea salt

1 teaspoon freshly ground black pepper

8 100% whole wheat slider buns

1 cup spring mix lettuce

1 large Roma tomato, sliced into 8 slices

Keep an Open Mind

Are you constantly burning your favorite foods on the grill? Leaving a grill's top open allows for more oxygen to circulate throughout the racks. Not only does this promote a more even cooking process, but the chances of burning your meat are much slimmer.

1. Over medium heat, sauté onions and minced garlic in 2 tablespoons of water until soft. Remove from heat and allow to cool.

2. Preheat grill to medium heat and prepare with olive oil spray.

3. Combine sautéed onions and ground turkey breast in a large mixing bowl with salt and pepper, and mix thoroughly.

4. Form turkey mixture into 8 similarly sized patties.

5. Place patties on grill with lid open, and grill for 5 minutes on each side.

6. Remove patties when internal temperature reaches 165°F, place on buns, and garnish with lettuce and tomato slices.

PER SERVING Calories: 147 | Fat: 1.7 g | Protein: 16.6 g | Sodium: 458 mg | Fiber: 2.6 g | Carbohydrates: 16.7 g | Sugar: 3.4 g

Veggie Toss

Featuring important, vitamin-rich raw vegetables that are delicious and nutritious, this veggie assortment is a great option for a snack or party. Pair with the Delicious Veggie Dip.

INGREDIENTS | SERVES 12

1 cup broccoli florets
1 cup cauliflower florets
2 carrots, cut into 3" sticks
1 cup cherry tomatoes
2 cups of the Delicious Veggie Dip (see recipe)

1. On a plate or platter, arrange veggies in groups.

2. Place the dip in a small bowl in the center of the vegetable assortment.

PER SERVING Calories: 20 | Fat: 0.3 g | Protein: 2.4 g | Sodium: 24 mg | Fiber: 1 g | Carbohydrates: 4 g | Sugar: 2.3 g

Delicious Veggie Dip

Always perched right in the middle of the crudité arrangement is the infamous dip packed with fat and calories. Ditch the storebought dip and try this version, made with clean ingredients.

INGREDIENTS | SERVES 12

1 cup plain Greek-style yogurt
1 cup low-fat plain yogurt
2 tablespoons white vinegar
3 tablespoons dried dill
½ small white onion, minced finely
1 teaspoon freshly ground black pepper

1. Combine all ingredients in a covered mixing bowl.

2. Mix ingredients until blended thoroughly.

3. Refrigerate for 2 hours, and serve.

PER SERVING Calories: 24 | Fat: 0.4 g | Protein: 5 g | Sodium: 27 mg | Fiber: 0.2 g | Carbohydrates: 3.6 g | Sugar: 3 g

Chicken Nachos

"Healthy nachos" sounds like an oxymoron, but this recipe makes it a tasty reality. The yogurt and seasonings are the only things that come prepared. This delicious mix of ingredients provides a healthy plate of nachos that'll make any others seem like a waste of time . . . and calories.

INGREDIENTS | SERVES 12

24 Tasty Tortilla Chips (see recipe in this chapter)

1 cup Spicy Clean Refried Beans (see recipe in this chapter)

¾ cup Great Guacamole (see recipe in this chapter)

2 grilled boneless, skinless chicken breasts, torn into bite-sized pieces

1 cup low-fat yogurt

2 teaspoons cumin

1. Layer the chips evenly on a large dish.

2. Place dollops of the refried beans atop the tortilla chips.

3. Cover the refried beans with the Great Guacamole.

4. Combine the chicken breast, yogurt, and cumin and layer on top of the guacamole.

PER SERVING Calories: 123 | Fat: 4.8 g | Protein: 11 g | Sodium: 199 mg | Fiber: 2.2 g | Carbohydrates: 8.6 g | Sugar: 1.7 g

Spinach and Artichoke Dip

Ditching the fat- and sodium-laden ingredients, this delicious dip goes from diet pitfall to party pleaser! Serve with Tasty Tortilla Chips (see recipe in this chapter) for one amazing pairing!

INGREDIENTS | SERVES 12

2 cups torn spinach leaves

½ cup chopped water chestnuts

1 cup chopped artichoke hearts

2 cups nonfat yogurt

2 teaspoons dried mustard

1 tablespoon white vinegar

1 teaspoon freshly ground black pepper

1 teaspoon garlic powder

1. Combine all ingredients thoroughly in a covered dish, cover, and refrigerate.

2. Allow flavors to marry and dip to chill 1–2 hours, and serve.

PER SERVING Calories: 39 | Fat: 1.5 g | Protein: 2 g | Sodium: 40 mg | Fiber: 1 g | Carbohydrates: 5 g | Sugar: 2.3 g

Scrumptious Salsa

Salsa is so versatile—why not learn how to make it at home with fresh ingredients? After all, poor ingredients are packed into the storebought varieties: sugar, sodium, and preservatives.

INGREDIENTS | SERVES 8

2 avocados, peeled and chopped
½ large red onion, peeled and chopped
½ large red pepper, chopped
½ small jalapeño, chopped and seeded
2 garlic cloves, crushed
¼ cup freshly squeezed lime juice
3 tablespoons chopped cilantro
1 teaspoon chili powder
¼ cup olive oil

1. Combine all ingredients in a medium bowl.

2. Cover and refrigerate for 2–12 hours before serving.

PER SERVING Calories: 163 | Fat: 15 g | Protein: 2 g | Sodium: 9 mg | Fiber: 5 g | Carbohydrates: 8.6 g | Sugar: 1.4 g

Melon Mix-Up

Sometimes eating fruit by itself gets boring. Jazz up your melons with aromatic and flavorful ginger!

INGREDIENTS | SERVES 4

½ cantaloupe
½ honeydew melon
2 tablespoons fresh ginger, grated
2 tablespoons freshly squeezed lemon juice
2 tablespoons agave nectar

1. Remove rind and seeds from melons, and cut into bite-sized pieces.

2. Combine the cantaloupe and honeydew in a medium casserole dish.

3. Sprinkle the grated ginger, agave, and the lemon juice atop the melon.

4. Toss to coat, refrigerate until chilled.

PER SERVING Calories: 103 | Fat: 0.3 g | Protein: 1.4 g | Sodium: 34 mg | Fiber: 1.8 g | Carbohydrates: 26 g | Sugar: 24 g

Great Guacamole

Full of flavor and "good-for-you" fats, this chunky dip is filling and nutritious. Beautiful colors from all the fresh ingredients make this delectable delight a feast for your eyes and your taste buds!

INGREDIENTS | SERVES 12

3 avocados, mashed to desired consistency

½ red onion, chopped

2 Roma tomatoes, chopped

2 tablespoons chopped cilantro

1 garlic clove, crushed

¼ cup freshly squeezed lime juice

1 teaspoon all-natural sea salt

1 teaspoon freshly ground black pepper

1. Combine all ingredients in a small mixing bowl and blend thoroughly.

2. Add salt and pepper to taste.

3. Serve immediately.

PER SERVING Calories: 84 | Fat: 7.4 g | Protein: 1.2 g | Sodium: 200 mg | Fiber: 3.6 g | Carbohydrates: 5.3 g | Sugar: 0.8 g

Avocados: Nature's Best Form of Healthy Fat

This fruit, a member of the pear family, is not only rich in vitamins and minerals—it's also packed with healthy fats that multitask for your body. Plentiful in vitamins A, C, and E, avocados are great for improving the performance of the brain and digestive system, and the body's metabolism of nutrients. The added benefits of strong and shiny skin, hair, and nails are just added bonuses to indulging in these great fresh fruits.

Spicy Clean Refried Beans

Refried beans get a bad rap because most storebought versions are high in fat or sodium. Amazingly rich in protein, nutrients, and vitamins, this healthy version of the sinful favorite allows you to enjoy a great snack with no guilt.

INGREDIENTS | SERVES 12

2½ cups dried pinto beans (soaked 12–24 hours)

4 tablespoons olive oil, divided

1 tablespoon chipotle powder

1 tablespoon cayenne pepper

2 teaspoons cumin

1 teaspoon onion powder

1 teaspoon garlic powder

½ teaspoon paprika

All-natural sea salt and freshly ground black pepper to taste

1. Combine soaked beans, 2 tablespoons of the olive oil, chipotle powder, cayenne pepper, cumin, onion powder, garlic powder, and paprika in a food processor or blender and blend until thoroughly combined.

2. Gradually add remaining 2 tablespoons of olive oil until desired consistency is achieved.

3. Add salt and pepper to taste.

PER SERVING Calories: 183 | Fat: 5 g | Protein: 8.7 g | Sodium: 6 mg | Fiber: 6.4 g | Carbohydrates: 26 g | Sugar: 1 g

Divine Deviled Eggs

Cleaning up the classic party favorites can be challenging . . . but it can be done! With this deliciously lightened-up version, you can enjoy eggs for the protein-packed super-morsels they truly are!

INGREDIENTS | SERVES 12

6 eggs, hard-boiled, cooled, and peeled

½ cup low-fat plain yogurt

1 stalk of celery, finely minced

1 teaspoon garlic powder

1 teaspoon onion powder

1 teaspoon freshly ground black pepper

Paprika, for garnish

1. Halve the eggs lengthwise, and remove yolks to a mixing bowl.

2. Mash the yolks, and mix with the yogurt, celery, garlic powder, onion powder, and black pepper.

3. Spoon the mixture into each of the egg white halves until filled and slightly bulging.

4. Sprinkle the eggs with paprika, cover, and refrigerate until ready to serve.

PER SERVING Calories: 44 | Fat: 2.6 g | Protein: 5 g | Sodium: 45 mg | Fiber: 0.1 g | Carbohydrates: 1.3 g | Sugar: 1 g

Best-Ever Bean Dip

*So many people avoid this popular party favorite because of heavy creams and cheeses.
Try this version instead at your next get-together. And, this is a great recipe
to serve with the Tasty Tortilla Chips (see recipe in this chapter).*

INGREDIENTS | SERVES 12

2 cups Spicy Clean Refried Beans (see recipe in this chapter)

1½ cups plain low-fat yogurt

1½ cups plain low-fat Greek-style yogurt

2 cups Scrumptious Salsa (see recipe in this chapter)

1 cup green onions, chopped

1 large tomato, chopped

2½ cups shredded lettuce

1 cup natural black olives, sliced

1. In a mixing bowl, combine the yogurt and Greek-style yogurt.

2. In a glass pie plate, layer the refried beans evenly for the bottom of the dip.

3. Top beans with ½ of the yogurt mix, followed by all of the salsa.

4. Top the salsa layer with the green onions, tomatoes, and lettuce.

5. Complete the dip with a layer of the remaining yogurt mix spread, and top with the sliced olives.

PER SERVING Calories: 97 | Fat: 2.3 g | Protein: 6 g | Sodium: 576 mg | Fiber: 3.5 g | Carbohydrates: 15 g | Sugar: 6.6 g

Easy Omelets

With all the hype about breakfast being the most important meal of the day, why confine energy-supplying breakfast ingredients to morning meals? Eggs are just as delicious as a snack!

INGREDIENTS | SERVES 2

4 eggs
2 tablespoons filtered water
½ cup chopped baby spinach leaves
2 tablespoons goat cheese

1. Prepare a small omelet-sized skillet with olive oil spray.

2. In a small bowl, beat eggs and water.

3. Over medium-high heat, wilt half of the spinach lightly.

4. Pour half of the egg mixture over spinach.

5. Using a spatula, pull edges into center, spreading spinach evenly throughout eggs.

6. Once center begins to bubble (about 2–3 minutes), wiggle the spatula under the omelet and turn over completely.

7. Continue cooking second side for 3–4 minutes until center is set and no juices remain.

8. Turn omelet over to original side and place half of goat cheese on one side, and fold over the other side to cover. Remove from heat and plate.

9. Repeat for second omelet.

PER SERVING Calories: 169 | Fat: 12 g | Protein: 14 g | Sodium: 250 mg | Fiber: 0.2 g | Carbohydrates: 1.5 g | Sugar: 1.2 g

Tuna Salad–Stuffed Tomatoes

You've probably heard of stuffed peppers—now give stuffed tomatoes a try! Overflowing with delicious tuna salad made from heart-healthy ingredients and flavorful spices, this delicious pairing of tasty salad and edible bowl makes for a protein-packed power snack!

INGREDIENTS | SERVES 6

1 can solid white albacore tuna, packed in water

½ cup plain low-fat yogurt

¼ cup chopped celery

¼ cup finely minced onion

1 teaspoon garlic powder

1 teaspoon all-natural sea salt, or to taste

1 teaspoon freshly ground black pepper

6 Roma tomatoes, tops and seeds removed

1. In a large mixing bowl, crush the drained tuna.

2. Add ½ cup of the low-fat yogurt, celery, onion, and garlic powder. Taste and add salt and pepper as needed.

3. Fill each cleaned tomato with ⅙ of the tuna mixture.

PER SERVING Calories: 92 | Fat: 3 g | Protein: 10.6 g | Sodium: 523 mg | Fiber: 1 g | Carbohydrates: 6 g | Sugar: 4 g

Benefits of Omega-Rich Snacks

When your brain starts feeling foggy and your focus is a little hazy, reaching for an omega-rich snack is your best option. Containing the healthy fats, rich fish like tuna can work wonders for your brain and your body. Not only do the omegas help your brain functioning, the protein in every bite helps your body run optimally and your belly feel full. Talk about multitasking!

Loaded Potato Skins

This delicious treat can be a scrumptious starter or a satisfying snack. Best of all, it has much less fat than you see in restaurant versions.

INGREDIENTS | SERVES 12

6 Idaho potatoes, baked

1 cup plain low-fat yogurt

1 cup Spicy Clean Refried Beans (see recipe in this chapter)

½ cup chopped chives

½ cup diced tomatoes

½ cup sliced olives

1. Preheat oven to 350°F. Slice baked potatoes in half lengthwise, and remove center, leaving ⅛"–¼" next to skin.

2. Layer the skins (flesh-side up) on a foil-lined baking sheet. Bake for 10–15 minutes, or until edges are slightly crispy.

3. Layer 1–2 tablespoons of the refried beans on each potato skin.

4. Top the beans with 1–2 tablespoons of the yogurt, and sprinkle the chives and tomatoes on top.

5. Garnish with the sliced olives.

PER SERVING Calories: 123 | Fat: 1.2 g | Protein: 4.6 g | Sodium: 157 mg | Fiber: 2.7 g | Carbohydrates: 24 g | Sugar: 2.4 g

Spicy Jalapeño Poppers

Sometimes it's the fried favorites that cause the worst cravings. Believe it or not, your cravings can be satisfied with clean alternatives. Introducing a heart-healthy, yet very delicious, recipe for jalapeño poppers that will make anyone's heart (and taste buds!) sing.

INGREDIENTS | SERVES 12

1 cup low-fat plain Greek-style yogurt
½ red onion, minced
½ cup tomatoes, minced
2 tablespoons garlic, minced
1 teaspoon all-natural sea salt
12 jalapeño peppers
1 cup almond milk
1 cup 100% whole wheat flour
½ cup olive oil

1. In a mixing bowl, combine yogurt, onion, tomatoes, garlic, and salt.

2. Remove tops and seeds from jalapeños, and stuff with the yogurt mixture.

3. Pour almond milk into a shallow dish next to a shallow dish filled with the whole wheat flour.

4. Dip each jalapeño into the almond milk and roll in the flour; set aside.

5. Heat the olive oil in a large skillet over medium heat. Add the jalapeños, turning regularly, and cook until golden brown all over.

6. Remove from oil and place onto paper towels to soak up excess oil.

PER SERVING Calories: 141 | Fat: 9.6 g | Protein: 3 g | Sodium: 218 mg | Fiber: 2 g | Carbohydrates: 12 g | Sugar: 3 g

Garlic and Herb Tortilla Chips

*These crunchy chips are great by themselves or paired with a delicious dip
like the Spicy Clean Refried Beans or Spinach and Artichoke Dip.*

INGREDIENTS | SERVES 10

4 100% whole wheat tortillas

1 teaspoon all-natural sea salt

2 teaspoons garlic powder

2 teaspoons sodium-free Italian
seasoning

1. Preheat oven to 350°F. Cut each tortilla into 8 pizza-shaped slices.

2. Line a baking sheet with aluminum foil and spray with olive oil spray.

3. Arrange the tortilla pieces evenly on the baking sheet, spray with olive oil, and sprinkle with the salt, garlic powder, and Italian seasoning.

4. Bake for 10–15 minutes, or until crispy.

PER SERVING Calories: 39 | Fat: 1 g |
Protein: 1 g | Sodium: 312 mg | Fiber: 0.4 g |
Carbohydrates: 6.5 g | Sugar: 0.2 g

Peppy Pesto

*Tons of recipes involve pesto, so have this version on hand! Keep it in
the refrigerator for 2–3 days, or in the freezer for up to 1 month.*

**INGREDIENTS | YIELDS 3 CUPS; SERVING
SIZE ¼ CUP**

2 cups baby spinach leaves, washed and
dried

1 cup fresh basil leaves, washed and
dried

½ cup toasted unsalted pine nuts

6 garlic cloves, peeled

2 tablespoons lemon juice

1 cup extra-virgin olive oil, divided

1 teaspoon all-natural sea salt

1 teaspoon freshly ground black pepper

1. In a food processor, combine the spinach, basil, pine nuts, garlic cloves, lemon juice, and ¼ cup of the olive oil. Process until well blended.

2. Drizzle remaining olive oil until desired consistency is achieved.

3. Add sea salt and pepper to taste.

PER SERVING Calories: 223 | Fat: 23.75 g |
Protein: 1.42 g | Sodium: 208.5 mg | Fiber: 1.25 g |
Carbohydrates: 2.83 g | Sugar: 0.1 g

Tasty Tomato Sauce

Homemade tomato sauce doesn't have to involve spending all day stirring a giant pot. Try this simple recipe, which uses fresh ingredients and savory spices, to create an amazing sauce that's free of preservatives and poor ingredients usually found in the storebought varieties.

INGREDIENTS | YIELDS 8 CUPS; SERVING SIZE 1 CUP

2 yellow onions, chopped

2 green bell peppers, chopped

1 tablespoon olive oil

8 large tomatoes, peeled and crushed

2 tablespoons minced garlic

6-ounce can organic tomato paste

1 teaspoon dried basil

1 teaspoon dried oregano

1 teaspoon Sucanat

2 teaspoons all-natural sea salt

2 teaspoons freshly ground black pepper

1. In a large skillet over medium heat, sauté the onions and green peppers in the olive oil until softened.

2. In a large pot over medium-low heat, combine the tomatoes (and their juice), sautéed onions and peppers, garlic, tomato paste, basil, and oregano. Stir the sauce and cover.

3. Simmer the sauce for about an hour.

4. Add the Sucanat, sea salt, and pepper to taste and stir.

PER SERVING Calories: 88.625 | Fat: 2.25 g | Protein: 3.25 g | Sodium: 767 mg | Fiber: 4.25 g | Carbohydrates: 16.625 g | Sugar: 9.75 g

Freeze Large Batches

Save time and energy by preparing one large batch of this delicious sauce and storing it in separate containers. It can be frozen for up to 3 months! This plan-ahead technique makes for a slew of quick dinners any day of the week!

"Good Gracious!" Granola

Rather than purchasing storebought granola that might have preservatives, trans fats, and other poor ingredients, whip up a delicious batch. Healthy, delicious, and packed with energy-boosting ingredients, this recipe is great mixed in with yogurt or as a crunchy topping on ice cream!

INGREDIENTS | YIELDS 10 CUPS; SERVING SIZE IS ½ CUP

½ cup all-natural organic maple syrup

½ cup natural organic honey

½ cup canola oil

1 teaspoon vanilla extract

8 cups natural rolled oats

1 cup toasted, unsalted sunflower seeds

1 cup natural pecans, measured then chopped

1 cup natural walnuts, measured then chopped

1 teaspoon cinnamon

2 cups honey wheat germ

1. Preheat the oven to 325°F, and prepare a baking sheet with aluminum foil and olive oil spray.

2. In a large mixing bowl, combine the syrup, honey, oil, and vanilla, and mix well.

3. Add the oats, sunflower seeds, chopped nuts, cinnamon, and wheat germ. Toss to coat evenly.

4. Spread the mixture on the prepared baking sheet, and bake for 15 minutes. Shake the mixture or turn with a spatula, return to the oven, and continue baking for 10–15 minutes, or until crispy.

PER SERVING Calories: 369.75 | Fat: 20.1 g | Protein: 9.8 g | Sodium: 4.85 mg | Fiber: 6.4 g | Carbohydrates: 41.25 g | Sugar: 10.9 g

Fruit Salsa

Delicious alone or paired with Cinnamon Chips, this delicious salsa was the idea of a wonderful friend, Arlene Brown, to whom I will be eternally grateful. Use fresh fruit for the best results, and prepare to enjoy a sensational delight.

INGREDIENTS | SERVES 12

1 cup chopped strawberries

1 cup chopped mango

1 cup chopped pineapple

2 kiwis, peeled and chopped

2 tablespoons chopped fresh mint

¼ cup freshly squeezed lime juice

Splendid Strawberries

Rich in antioxidants and packed with more than 100 percent of your daily value of vitamin C, strawberries are not only delicious, but nutritious. The leading antioxidants in these berries are anthocyanins, which play a major role in protecting the body from free radicals that can damage cells.

Combine all fruit with mint and lime juice in a covered container. Chill for 1 hour.

PER SERVING Calories: 28 | Fat: 0.1 g | Protein: 0.3 g | Sodium: 1.4 mg | Fiber: 1.2 g | Carbohydrates: 7 g | Sugar: 3.9 g

CHAPTER 5

Simple Sandwiches and Wraps

Tempting Tilapia and Veggie Wraps

Don't think of fish as only a dinnertime meal! This beautiful combination of delicious and nutritious fish and vegetables rolls up quickly in a filling whole wheat tortilla.

INGREDIENTS | SERVES 2

1 small onion, sliced in strips

1 yellow squash, sliced

1 zucchini, sliced

2 tablespoons olive oil, divided

2 garlic cloves, crushed

1 lemon, juiced

2 100% whole wheat tortillas

1 pound tilapia fillet

1 teaspoon all-natural sea salt

1 teaspoon freshly ground black pepper

The Whole Truth on Whole Wheat

The guidelines in the United States for labeling wheat products as such require manufacturers to use only 60 percent of the whole wheat berry. This means that the 40 percent that was removed was replaced and enriched with undesirable ingredients and additives that make for a bread that's not the healthy version you think it might be. By choosing wheat products that state "100 percent whole wheat," you can be sure that the bran and the germ of the wheat (the most beneficial parts) remain in your food.

1. Over medium heat, prepare a large skillet with olive oil spray.

2. Add onion slices, squash, and zucchini, and drizzle with 1 tablespoon of the olive oil. Sauté for 4–5 minutes, then add crushed garlic and half of the lemon juice. Continue sautéing for 5 minutes, or until all vegetables are slightly softened.

3. Remove vegetables from the heat and place equal servings in mounds on the two tortillas.

4. Return skillet to medium heat and drizzle with remaining tablespoon of olive oil.

5. Rinse tilapia fillet and place in heated skillet with the rest of the lemon juice.

6. Allow fillet to cook undisturbed for 3–5 minutes or until fish begins to whiten through.

7. Flip fillet and continue cooking for 5 minutes, or until fish is flaky and no juices remain.

8. Remove fish from heat, crumble or halve, and place atop each vegetable mound with salt and pepper to taste.

PER SERVING Calories: 453 | Fat: 18 g | Protein: 45 g | Sodium: 1,000 mg | Fiber: 4 g | Carbohydrates: 28 g | Sugar: 7 g

Marvelous Mediterranean Wraps

Skip the preservative-packed frozen lunch and opt for this cleaned-up version instead!
Brimming with healthy ingredients, vitamins, and health benefits, this is a
light lunch that will taste great and make you feel great, too!

INGREDIENTS | SERVES 2

4 tablespoons plain low-fat Greek-style yogurt

1 grilled boneless, skinless chicken breast, torn into bite-sized pieces

½ cup homemade sun-dried tomatoes (see sidebar)

½ cup roasted red peppers

½ cup sliced olives

½ cup artichoke hearts, chopped

1 teaspoon garlic powder

1 teaspoon all-natural sea salt

2 100% whole wheat tortillas

1. In a mixing bowl, combine the yogurt, chicken, sun-dried tomatoes, red peppers, olives, artichokes, and garlic powder. Add salt to taste.

2. Lay tortillas on a flat surface and spoon half of the mixture down the center of each wrap.

3. Wrap tightly and enjoy!

PER SERVING Calories: 352 | Fat: 9 g | Protein: 33 g | Sodium: 1587 mg | Fiber: 6 g | Carbohydrates: 35 g | Sugar: 10 g

Homemade Sun-Dried Tomatoes

To make about 10 servings of sun-dried tomatoes, line a baking sheet with foil and preheat oven to 200°F. Quarter 5 plum tomatoes and arrange on the baking sheet. Drizzle with 1 tablespoon extra-virgin olive oil and sprinkle with 1 teaspoon no-salt Italian seasoning, 1 teaspoon garlic powder, and 1 teaspoon all-natural sea salt. Bake for 8 hours.

Spinach, Chicken, and Goat Cheese Wraps

When you're stuck in a middle-of-the-day funk, the last thing you need is a heavy fast-food lunch to weigh you down. Instead, try this delicious light lunch wrap. You'll feel full, but you won't need a nap after you eat!

INGREDIENTS | SERVES 2

2 100% whole wheat tortillas

2 tablespoons plain Greek-style yogurt

1 cup baby spinach leaves, measured then chopped

1 grilled boneless, skinless chicken breast, torn into bite-sized pieces

½ cup crumbled goat cheese

2 teaspoons red wine vinegar

1. Lay tortillas on a flat surface and spoon 1 tablespoon of the yogurt down the center of each wrap.

2. Layer the chopped spinach leaves on top of the yogurt.

3. Top with even portions of the torn chicken and crumbled goat cheese.

4. Drizzle 1 teaspoon of the red wine vinegar on each mound of food, wrap tightly, and enjoy!

PER SERVING Calories: 337 | Fat: 13 g | Protein: 33 g | Sodium: 766 mg | Fiber: 1.3 g | Carbohydrates: 18 g | Sugar: 3 g

The Many Benefits of Spinach

Popeye wasn't that far off in his obsession with spinach for great health. Not only does this amazing leafy green count for important daily vegetable servings, the amount of vitamins and minerals in every healthy bunch makes spinach one of the most nutrient-dense food options available. Rich in iron, an important mineral for blood health, spinach is worth its weight in gold when it comes to your health . . . and taste!

Curry Chicken Gyros

Gyros from a food cart or local restaurant may come with great flavor, but you're also getting plenty of fat, calories, and sodium, too! This gyro, on the other hand, uses all fresh ingredients. The light cucumber dressing adds a refreshing dimension.

INGREDIENTS | SERVES 2

1 boneless, skinless chicken breast, chopped

½ yellow onion, minced

1 tablespoon olive oil

½ teaspoon garlic powder

½ teaspoon dried thyme

½ teaspoon dried marjoram

½ teaspoon dried basil

½ teaspoon dried oregano

½ cup cucumber, peeled and thinly sliced

½ cup plain Greek-style yogurt

1 tablespoon lime juice

1 tablespoon fresh dill

2 100% whole wheat pita rounds

2 cups shredded lettuce

½ tomato, cut into 4 slices

2 tablespoons crumbled goat cheese

1. In a large skillet, sauté the chicken and onions together in the olive oil and seasonings until cooked through, and remove from heat.

2. In a small dish, combine the sliced cucumber, yogurt, lime juice, and dill.

3. Place the pitas on a flat surface and spoon the chicken and onions down the center of each.

4. Cover the chicken with the cucumber yogurt dressing, and top with the lettuce, tomato, and goat cheese.

5. Roll tightly and serve.

PER SERVING Calories: 353 | Fat: 13 g | Protein: 32 g | Sodium: 493 mg | Fiber: 2.5 g | Carbohydrates: 26 g | Sugar: 8 g

Spices That Do More Than Add Flavor

Certain spices like cayenne, turmeric, curry, and cumin have been shown to increase metabolism and promote healthier functioning of the body's systems in numerous studies performed at the University of Chicago. By adding a sprinkling of this or a pinch of that, you can optimize your health while making your food taste great.

Too-Good Turkey Burgers

While you want to skip the fast-food hamburgers for lunch, that doesn't mean that all burgers are bad for you. These turkey burgers give you a great protein boost without the fat and sodium you'll find at restaurants.

INGREDIENTS | SERVES 4

1 pound ground turkey breast

1 teaspoon minced garlic

½ cup chopped onions

1 teaspoon all-natural sea salt

1 teaspoon freshly ground black pepper

1 cup shredded romaine hearts

4 slices beefsteak tomato

4 100% whole wheat hamburger buns

High-Fructose Corn Syrup in Breads

While hamburger buns' packaging may ensure that they're 100% whole wheat, read the ingredient list anyway. Make sure that whole wheat flour is the first ingredient listed, then look for high-fructose corn syrup, which can cause a nasty sugar crash. Choose foods without this highly processed ingredient and opt for natural sweeteners instead.

1. Prepare a grill with olive oil spray and heat to medium heat.

2. Prepare a sauté pan with olive oil spray over medium heat, and add onions. Sauté until soft and translucent.

3. In a large mixing bowl, add the ground turkey breast, minced garlic, sautéed onions, salt, and pepper, and combine thoroughly. Form into 4 patties of the same size.

4. Place patties on the open grill's flame, and cook for 5–7 minutes undisturbed.

5. Flip the patties and continue cooking for 5–7 minutes, or until juices run clear.

6. Open the buns, and move each patty to the bottom half of each bun.

7. Top burgers with the sliced tomato, shredded lettuce, and bun top, and enjoy!

PER SERVING Calories: 225 | Fat: 2.5 g | Protein: 30 g | Sodium: 754 mg | Fiber: 2.8 g | Carbohydrates: 19 g | Sugar: 2.7 g

Lean, Mean Sloppy Joes

Forget about the school lunchroom sloppy joes, with mystery meat and questionable taste. Rediscovery why this sandwich is an American favorite by using this clean recipe!

INGREDIENTS | SERVES 6

1 tablespoon olive oil

1 onion, minced

1 green pepper, minced

1 pound organic lean ground beef

1 egg

½ teaspoon garlic powder

1½ teaspoons dry mustard

1 teaspoon Worcestershire sauce

3 tablespoons filtered water

6 100% whole wheat hamburger buns

Why Organic Beef Is Better

While some say that the focus on organic products is all hype, others disagree. Antibiotics, steroids, and hormones have become a hazardous reality in nonorganic beef; buying organic beef products ensures that your meat will be free of these undesirable additives.

1. In a large skillet over medium heat, drizzle the olive oil and sauté the onion and pepper until soft.

2. In a large mixing bowl, combine the beef, egg, sautéed onion and green pepper, garlic powder, mustard, and Worcestershire, and mix until thoroughly combined.

3. Return the mixture to the skillet and continue to cook over medium heat, stirring constantly.

4. If the meat seems to be drying out before completely done, add water 1 tablespoon at a time, and continue cooking until the mixture has your preference of the perfect sloppy joe consistency and all meat is browned.

5. Remove from heat and scoop six even servings onto each of the whole wheat buns.

PER SERVING Calories: 214 | Fat: 7 g | Protein: 19 g | Sodium: 257 mg | Fiber: 1.3 g | Carbohydrates: 15 g | Sugar: 2.5 g

The Perfect CLT Sandwiches

Sure, you might see BLTs more often on menus—but CLTs are a much cleaner choice! Skip the fatty bacon and enjoy this flavorful sandwich instead.

INGREDIENTS | SERVES 2

2 boneless, skinless chicken breasts
1 teaspoon garlic powder
Freshly ground black pepper
1 teaspoon Italian seasoning
1 teaspoon balsamic vinegar
1 cup shredded romaine hearts
2 slices beefsteak tomato
2 100% whole wheat hamburger buns

The Breakdown on Bacon

While bacon may be a traditional favorite for breakfasts and some club sandwiches, the truth is that it's better to opt for other healthier items on the menu. Pork bacon, turkey bacon, low-sodium, and low-fat varieties really only make slight improvements on the same, less-than-ideal product. High in saturated fat, sodium, additives, preservatives, and more, bacon should be an occasional treat rather than a frequent staple.

1. Prepare a grill with olive oil spray over medium heat.

2. Sprinkle garlic powder, black pepper, and Italian seasoning on the breasts, and place on the open grill's flames.

3. Cook the breasts for 7–8 minutes, turn, and continue cooking for another 7 minutes, or until juices run clear.

4. While the breasts finish, dash the balsamic vinegar over the chicken.

5. Remove the breasts from the grill, and place onto buns.

6. Top chicken with tomato slices, shredded lettuce, and bun top.

PER SERVING Calories: 347 | Fat: 7 g | Protein: 52 g | Sodium: 447 mg | Fiber: 1.4 g | Carbohydrates: 15 g | Sugar: 1.9 g

Wacky Waldorf Wraps

Sometimes you need more than a salad to get you through a busy day. Here's the perfect solution—all the great tastes of a Waldorf salad, with the benefit of a filling wrap! Sweet and crunchy, this delicious mix is a tempting snack or meal for any time of day!

INGREDIENTS | SERVES 2

½ red apple, minced
½ cup chopped celery
½ cup grapes, quartered
½ cup walnuts, crushed
2 tablespoons plain nonfat yogurt
1 teaspoon nutmeg
2 100% whole wheat tortilla wraps

1. In a mixing bowl, combine the minced apple, celery, grapes, walnuts, yogurt, and nutmeg, and blend well.

2. Lay the tortillas flat, and spoon half of the mixture down the center of each wrap.

3. Wrap tightly, and enjoy!

PER SERVING Calories: 331 | Fat: 21 g | Protein: 7 g | Sodium: 223 mg | Fiber: 4 g | Carbohydrates: 32 g | Sugar: 13 g

Chicken Salad Pitas

This deliciously light favorite is cleaned up, packed with protein, and features fresh veggies and aromatic seasonings that allow for a drastic reduction in sodium. Enjoy this healthy version for a snack on its own or with bread as a delicious sandwich.

INGREDIENTS | SERVES 2

2 100% whole wheat pita halves
2 cups cooked boneless, skinless chicken breast, torn
½ cup low-fat plain yogurt
½ cup chopped celery
½ cup minced onion
1 teaspoon garlic powder
1 teaspoon freshly ground black pepper
1 teaspoon all-natural sea salt

1. Open pita halves.

2. In a mixing bowl, add chicken, yogurt, celery, onion, and seasonings, and mix until thoroughly combined.

3. Spoon half of chicken salad mixture into each pita.

PER SERVING Calories: 372 | Fat: 7 g | Protein: 50 g | Sodium: 995 mg | Fiber: 2.2 g | Carbohydrates: 24 g | Sugar: 7 g

Zippy Zucchini Stacked Sandwiches

Tangy sautéed zucchini slices meets creamy goat cheese for a fresh sandwich that will jump-start any midday slump. Light, yet satisfying, this simple low-calorie lunch is a perfect pick-me-up!

INGREDIENTS | SERVES 2

4 slices sprouted grain bread
1 large zucchini
1 tablespoon balsamic vinegar
2 tablespoons crumbled goat cheese

Zucchini: A Blank Canvas for Flavor

Zucchini is a nutritious vegetable that's packed with powerful vitamins and minerals (such as magnesium, potassium, manganese, and vitamins A and C) and lots of water. Because the taste can be a little "blank," this is the perfect food to spice up in any way you choose. Adding very strong flavors to zucchini will only solidify the spices' flavors, not contradict the flavor of the zucchini. Besides balsamic vinegar, try bold choices such as delicious herbs like basil, rosemary, or cilantro and other vinegar varieties.

1. Prepare a skillet with olive oil spray over medium heat.

2. Cut the zucchini in half, and slice thin lengthwise slices.

3. Arrange the zucchini slices in the skillet and cook for 3 minutes, turning frequently.

4. Sprinkle the slices with the balsamic vinegar and continue cooking until slightly soft. Remove from heat.

5. Lay two slices of the bread on two plates. Sprinkle ¼ of the goat cheese on each slice and cover each with half of the zucchini slices.

6. Sprinkle half of the remaining goat cheese on each sandwich and cover with remaining bread.

PER SERVING Calories: 192 | Fat: 4 g | Protein: 7 g | Sodium: 459 mg | Fiber: 2.8 g | Carbohydrates: 32 g | Sugar: 7.7 g

Blackened Mahi-Mahi Sandwiches

Amazingly flavorful, this mahi-mahi sandwich may be the fish-lover's clean dream for lunchtime. An easy way to get those twice-weekly recommended fish servings, this is sure to be one of your go-to recipes for a quick fish dish.

INGREDIENTS | SERVES 2

1 teaspoon cayenne pepper

1 teaspoon paprika

1 teaspoon cumin

1 teaspoon freshly ground black pepper

1 teaspoon all-natural sea salt

1 teaspoon onion powder

2 mahi-mahi fillets (about 1 pound), rinsed

4 slices sprouted grain bread

1 cup shredded romaine hearts

2 slices beefsteak tomato

2 tablespoons plain nonfat yogurt

¼ cup freshly squeezed lime juice

1 tablespoon chopped mint

Blackened Spice Rubs Made Healthy

Because fish is healthy on its own, *keeping it healthy when you cook it only makes sense.* But prepackaged blackening or store-bought seasonings can add loads of sodium or empty calories to a dish that needs only a little spice to do the trick. Making your own spicy combination at home is the healthiest way. Mix the spices listed here for your very own homemade blackening seasoning.

1. Prepare a large skillet over medium heat with olive oil spray.

2. Mix the cayenne, paprika, cumin, pepper, salt, and onion powder in a shallow dish and completely coat fish on both sides by dredging them in the spice mix.

3. Place the fillets on the hot skillet and cook for 4–5 minutes on each side or until crispy and flaky.

4. Place the two fillets on two separate slices of the bread, and top with the shredded lettuce and tomato.

5. In a small mixing bowl, combine the yogurt, lime juice, and mint, and spread half of the mixture on each piece of bread intended to top the sandwiches, and cover.

PER SERVING Calories: 176 | Fat: 2.3 g | Protein: 32 g | Sodium: 1140 mg | Fiber: 2 g | Carbohydrates: 5.4 g | Sugar: 1.8 g

Sweet and Spicy Chicken Wraps

Freshly squeezed orange juice sweetens this spicy wrapped-up chicken delight in a zesty way!

INGREDIENTS | SERVES 2

¼ cup low-fat plain Greek-style yogurt

¼ cup freshly squeezed orange juice

2 teaspoons freshly grated orange zest

2 teaspoons red pepper flakes

1 grilled boneless, skinless chicken breast, torn into bite-sized pieces

2 100% whole wheat tortillas

1. In a mixing bowl, combine the yogurt, orange juice, orange zest, and red pepper flakes.

2. Fold chicken in the yogurt mixture until well-blended.

3. Lay tortillas flat, and spoon ½ of the chicken mixture down the center of each tortilla.

4. Wrap tightly, and enjoy.

PER SERVING Calories: 208 | Fat: 4.5 g | Protein: 18.8 g | Sodium: 289 mg | Fiber: 1.6 g | Carbohydrates: 22 g | Sugar: 5.7 g

Tasty Turkey Avocado Wraps

This wrap is simple and quick, yet absolutely delicious.

INGREDIENTS | SERVES 2

4 ⅛"-thick slices of roasted turkey breast

1 avocado, skin and seed removed

2 100% whole wheat tortillas

2 tablespoons lemon juice

½ cup diced tomatoes

1 teaspoon chopped mint

Food Combining

Combine carbs, protein, and fat to ensure that your diet is well rounded and that your body is getting the nutrition it needs. Protein helps to repair muscles; carbohydrates aid in energy production; and fats promote better system functioning, especially in the brain.

1. Cut turkey breast slices into thin strips, separating into two equal servings.

2. Slice the avocado into thin strips.

3. Lay the tortillas flat and place each serving of the turkey breast down the center of each wrap. Lay the avocado slices over the turkey, and drizzle with the lemon juice.

4. Top the avocado with the diced tomato and mint, wrap tightly, and enjoy!

PER SERVING Calories: 358 | Fat: 18 g | Protein: 24 g | Sodium: 254 mg | Fiber: 8 g | Carbohydrates: 26 g | Sugar: 2.7 g

Shrimp Salsa Pitas

My wonderful Aunt Sue Deitz serves this amazing shrimp salad as a full lunch or as a delicious appetizer. Light, flavorful, and totally satisfying, this sweet and slightly spicy shrimp salad pita will excite your taste buds and give you a little bounce to your step.

INGREDIENTS | SERVES 2

½ pound steamed medium shrimp, chopped
½ cup chopped celery
½ cup chopped mango
½ cup chopped tomato
½ cup chopped red onion
½ cup chopped avocado
½ cup fresh lime juice
1 100% whole wheat pita, cut in half

1. In a mixing bowl, combine the shrimp, celery, mango, tomato, red onion, avocado, and lime juice, and mix well.

2. Spoon mixture into each pita half.

> **PER SERVING** Calories: 266 | Fat: 8 g | Protein: 25 g | Sodium: 282 mg | Fiber: 5 g | Carbohydrates: 23 g | Sugar: 10 g

Tomato, Mozzarella, and Basil Wraps

You've probably had these mouthwatering flavors in an appetizer before—fresh mozzarella paired with hearty tomatoes and aromatic basil. Try them in this wrap for an equally enjoyable option!

INGREDIENTS | SERVES 2

4 beefsteak tomato slices
2 ¼" slices of fresh mozzarella cheese
2 100% whole wheat tortillas
2 tablespoons balsamic vinegar
1 teaspoon freshly ground black pepper
4 tablespoons chopped fresh basil leaves

1. Cut tomato slices and cheese slices into thin strips.

2. Lay tortillas flat, and layer half of the mozzarella strips down the center of each tortilla, followed by the tomato slices on top.

3. Drizzle the balsamic vinegar and cracked black pepper over the mozzarella and tomato, and cover with the chopped basil.

4. Wrap tightly, and enjoy!

> **PER SERVING** Calories: 213.17 | Fat: 9.56 g | Protein: 10.10 g | Sodium: 212.63 mg | Fiber: 1.69 g | Carbohydrates: 21.08 g | Sugar: 4.35 g

Roasted Red Pepper and Zucchini Wraps

These wraps come together super-fast when you're looking for a light lunch.

INGREDIENTS | SERVES 2

1 roasted red pepper (see sidebar)
1 small zucchini, sliced
2 100% whole wheat tortillas
2 teaspoons balsamic vinegar
1 teaspoon freshly ground black pepper

Homemade Roasted Red Peppers

Rather than purchasing some of the nonorganic, sodium-laden varieties, you can instead prepare delicious roasted red peppers healthfully at home! Preheating your oven to broil, remove the tops and seeds from the peppers and cut into ¾" strips. Laying the strips on a foil-lined baking sheet with the shiny side facing up, coat each strip with extra-virgin olive oil, and broil until the strips begin to char. Remove from the oven, allow to cool, and remove charred bits.

1. Roast the zucchini and red peppers (see sidebar).

2. Lay tortillas flat, and set ½ of the red pepper strips down the center of each.

3. Top the red peppers with the roasted zucchini slices.

4. Drizzle the balsamic vinegar over the vegetables, and sprinkle the black pepper over top.

5. Wrap tortillas tightly, and enjoy!

PER SERVING Calories: 119 | Fat: 3 g | Protein: 4 g | Sodium: 198 mg | Fiber: 3 g | Carbohydrates: 20 g | Sugar: 3 g

Clean Tuna Salad Sandwiches

Normally packed with fattening mayonnaise, sugar, and sodium-laden relish, this classic needed a bit of a makeover before getting the clean thumbs-up. Now, you can enjoy this fabulous favorite with all the taste and none of the guilt.

INGREDIENTS | SERVES 2

1 can solid white albacore tuna in water

3 tablespoons plain nonfat yogurt

½ cup minced celery

1 teaspoon garlic powder

1 teaspoon onion powder

4 slices sprouted grain bread

1. Open the tuna, drain, and move to a mixing bowl.

2. Mash the tuna with a fork, then add the yogurt, celery, garlic powder, and onion powder. Mix well to combine thoroughly.

3. Spoon half of the mixture onto two of the bread slices, and top with the plain slices.

PER SERVING Calories: 329 | Fat: 9 g | Protein: 30 g | Sodium: 679 mg | Fiber: 2 g | Carbohydrates: 29 g | Sugar: 3.8 g

Canned Tuna Benefits

Adhering to the clean lifestyle can be made super-easy with canned tuna as an ingredient in many of your dishes. Solid white albacore tuna can be found in any grocery store, and provides valuable protein. While many people get concerned about mercury levels of certain fish like tuna, the canned variety that is solid white albacore has little risk in comparison to the "fresh" seafood market's available tuna steaks.

Thanksgiving on a Bun

What to do with all those Thanksgiving leftovers? Rather than duplicating your holiday meal, pack up those ingredients in this delicious sandwich for a quick, healthy, and satisfying way to use up what's left in your fridge. Or create it with other recipes from this book!

INGREDIENTS | SERVES 2

4 slices sprouted grain bread

4 slices ⅛"-thick roasted turkey breast (see recipe)

½ cup Mashed Potatoes and Cauliflower (see recipe in Chapter 15)

½ cup Clean Green Bean Casserole (see recipe in Chapter 15)

½ cup Better Than Classic Cranberry Sauce (see recipe in Chapter 15)

Multitasking Meals

When you're planning to make a big meal, try to anticipate what leftovers you'll have. Then, proactively plan a second meal around those leftovers. You'll save money by making that one meal stretch into two, and save time by already having some of the second meal's ingredients ready to go.

1. Set the bread slices out, and stack two slices of turkey breast on two of the slices.

2. Spread half of the mashed cauliflower over each sandwich's turkey breast slices.

3. Cover the cauliflower layer with the green bean casserole.

4. Spoon the cranberry sauce evenly over the two.

5. Close the sandwiches with the remaining two slices of bread, and enjoy!

PER SERVING Calories: 271 | Fat: 2.5 g | Protein: 32 g | Sodium: 491 mg | Fiber: 3 g | Carbohydrates: 28 g | Sugar: 2.8 g

Turkey Cranberry Wraps

This is a simple wrap that's delicious and bursting with flavor. It's simple to make, but it's an aromatic savory and sweet taste combination you're sure to enjoy!

INGREDIENTS | SERVES 2

2 100% whole wheat tortillas

4 ⅛" slices Spice-Rubbed Roasted Turkey Breast (see recipe in Chapter 6)

½ cup Better Than Classic Cranberry Sauce (see recipe in Chapter 15)

1. Cut turkey breast into strips, and place half down the center of each tortilla.

2. Cover the turkey strips with the cranberry sauce.

3. Wrap tightly, and enjoy!

PER SERVING Calories: 213.70 | Fat: 2.52 g | Protein: 6.07 g | Sodium: 217.74 mg | Fiber: 1.62 g | Carbohydrates: 42.34 g | Sugar: 26.82 g

Beans and Rice Wraps

Beans and rice isn't just a side dish anymore! In this recipe, it takes center stage as the perennial carb-and-protein match made in heaven. This is a great way to use up leftover beans.

INGREDIENTS | SERVES 2

2 100% whole wheat tortillas

½ cup Spicy Clean Refried Beans (see recipe in Chapter 4)

1 cup cooked brown rice

½ cup cooked black beans

½ cup cooked pinto beans

½ cup fresh kernel corn

1. Lay tortillas flat and spread half of the refried beans over each.

2. In a small mixing bowl, combine rice with beans and corn.

3. Spoon rice and beans mixture down the center of each tortilla, wrap tightly, and enjoy!

PER SERVING Calories: 402.49 | Fat: 5.02 g | Protein: 15.57 g | Sodium: 826.82 mg | Fiber: 13.02 g | Carbohydrates: 75.72 g | Sugar: 3.71 g

Spicy Chicken Burgers

You probably use ground beef and ground turkey frequently—but have you ever considered ground chicken breast? Look for it in your grocer's meat section.

INGREDIENTS | SERVES 6

1 pound organic ground chicken breast
½ roasted red pepper, minced
1 teaspoon onion powder
3 teaspoons red pepper flakes
4 slices beefsteak tomato
1 cup shredded romaine hearts
6 100% whole wheat hamburger buns

1. In a large mixing bowl, combine the ground chicken breast, roasted red pepper, onion powder, and red pepper flakes. Mix well, and form into six evenly sized burger patties.

2. Prepare a grill with olive oil spray over medium heat.

3. Place burgers on hot grill surface and cook for 5–7 minutes.

4. Flip burgers and continue cooking for 5–7 minutes, or until juices run clear.

5. Remove burgers from heat and set onto buns.

6. Top burgers with tomato slices, shredded lettuce, and bun tops.

PER SERVING Calories: 227.95 | Fat: 3.80 g | Protein: 20.12 g | Sodium: 429.25 mg | Fiber: 1.99 g | Carbohydrates: 27.35 g | Sugar: 2.95 g

Portabella Mushroom Burgers

Hearty portabella mushroom caps flavored with olive oil and aromatic spices get topped with roasted red peppers and goat cheese for a taste that will absolutely blow you away! Thanks to my wonderful Dad and Miss Pam for this delicious recipe!

INGREDIENTS | SERVES 2

2 large portabella mushroom caps
2 tablespoons olive oil
1 teaspoon garlic powder
1 teaspoon freshly ground black pepper
2 100% whole wheat hamburger buns
½ cup crumbled goat cheese
4 strips roasted red pepper

1. Prepare a grill with olive oil spray over medium heat.

2. Paint the underside of the mushroom caps with ¼ tablespoon of olive oil each. Sprinkle each cap with the garlic powder and black pepper.

3. Set the caps on the grill with the gills facing down, and paint the tops with remaining olive oil.

4. Grill for 4–6 minutes, flip, and continue grilling for 5 minutes.

5. Remove the mushrooms from the grill and set one on each bun bottom, with gills facing up.

6. Sprinkle gills with the crumbled goat cheese, and lay roasted red pepper strips on top.

7. Cover with bun tops and enjoy.

PER SERVING Calories: 579.20 | Fat: 34.99 g | Protein: 26.99 g | Sodium: 619.79 mg | Fiber: 3.54 g | Carbohydrates: 43.68 g | Sugar: 5.71 g

Grilled Chicken and Pineapple Sandwiches

This recipe is one sweet vacation from the normal boring everyday lunch break!

INGREDIENTS | SERVES 2

2 skinless, boneless chicken breasts
4 pineapple slices of ¼" thickness
½ cup freshly juiced pineapple juice
2 100% whole wheat buns

1. Prepare a grill with olive oil spray to medium heat.

2. Place the chicken breasts on the hot grill and pour ¼ cup of the pineapple juice over the breasts. Cook for 7 minutes.

3. Turn the breasts over, and pour the remaining pineapple juice over the breasts. Continue cooking for another 7 minutes or until juices run clear.

4. Place the pineapple slices on the grill and cook for 3 minutes before turning. Remove chicken and pineapple slices from the grill, stack on whole wheat buns, and enjoy!

PER SERVING Calories: 542 | Fat: 7 g | Protein: 54 g | Sodium: 412 mg | Fiber: 6.8 g | Carbohydrates: 65 g | Sugar: 41 g

CHAPTER 6

Marvelous Meats

Marvelous Meats (continued)

Garlic Chicken Stir-Fry

Stir-fries are the perfect quick meal when your family has rushed in from afternoon activities and everyone's starving. Serve over some brown rice if you like.

INGREDIENTS | SERVES 4

1 tablespoon olive oil

1 cup broccoli florets

1 yellow onion, quartered

1 cup carrot matchsticks

1 cup snow peas

1 cup white mushrooms, sliced

2 tablespoons minced garlic

4 tablespoons filtered water, divided

2 boneless, skinless chicken breasts, cut in 1" cubes

1 teaspoon all-natural sea salt

MSG in Takeout

Monosodium glutamate, otherwise known as MSG, is a powerful additive and flavor enhancer. In the late 1960s and early 1970s, people started referring to the effects of MSG as "Chinese Restaurant Syndrome," when people sometimes experienced headaches, tightness in the chest, feelings of weakness, and hot sensations shortly after eating takeout Chinese food. Even today, MSG is often used at restaurants, so it's much healthier to make your own stir-fries at home.

1. Heat olive oil in a large skillet or wok over medium heat.

2. Sauté broccoli, onion, carrots, snow peas, and mushrooms with the garlic and 2 tablespoons water.

3. Cover skillet and cook vegetables for three minutes. Uncover and continue cooking and tossing vegetables for 3 minutes.

4. Add chicken and remaining water to skillet.

5. Stir-fry mixture until the chicken is completely cooked through with juices running clear, about 6 minutes.

6. Sprinkle with salt, remove from heat, and enjoy!

PER SERVING Calories: 143.28 | Fat: 5.39 g | Protein: 14.43 g | Sodium: 662.89 mg | Fiber: 2.50 g | Carbohydrates: 9.88 g | Sugar: 3.88 g

Pork Loin and Roasted Root Vegetables

This recipe is great for the cooler or winter months. Roasted with nutrition-packed root vegetables, this perfect combination of protein and carbohydrates makes for a hearty and healthy dish!

INGREDIENTS | SERVES 4

4 Idaho potatoes

4 carrots, peeled and tops removed

2 yellow onions, skin removed

2 tablespoons olive oil

2 teaspoons all-natural sea salt, divided

2 teaspoons freshly ground black pepper, divided

2 teaspoons smoked paprika, divided

1 teaspoon turmeric

1 pound pork tenderloin

Pork: Still the Other White Meat

Pork's popularity seems to come and go—be sure you're giving it a chance! Low in fat and calories, plentiful in vitamins and nutrients such as thiamin, niacin, riboflavin, and vitamin B$_6$, pork is a great-tasting source of powerful protein. This delicious cut of meat can be enjoyed guilt-free in recipes that roast, bake, sauté, or grill!

1. Preheat oven to 400°F, and prepare a 9" x 13" baking dish with olive oil spray.

2. Cut potatoes, carrots, and onions in similar bite-sized pieces.

3. In a large resealable plastic bag, combine the potatoes, carrots, onions, and olive oil with 1 teaspoon of the salt, 1 teaspoon of the pepper, 1 teaspoon of the paprika, and the turmeric, and toss to coat evenly.

4. Pour the vegetables in an even layer in the prepared dish.

5. Cook at 400°F for 30 minutes.

6. Remove veggies from the oven, stir, and clear a space large enough to fit the pork tenderloin in the middle of the vegetables. Top the pork loin with the remaining spices.

7. Return the pan to the oven, and continue cooking at 400°F for 30–40 minutes, or until meat thermometer inserted in the center of the pork reads 165°F.

PER SERVING Calories: 388.29 | Fat: 9.86 g | Protein: 28.65 g | Sodium: 1304.12 mg | Fiber: 8.90 g | Carbohydrates: 47.20 g | Sugar: 8.34 g

Shepherd's Pie

This classic family favorite was begging for a clean makeover. This recipe's unique blend of spices and clean ingredients give you all the comforting flavor you love without the fat and calories you don't. Enjoy it tonight, then freeze the leftovers!

INGREDIENTS | SERVES 16

2 pounds browned ground turkey breast

1 onion, minced

4 teaspoons garlic powder

4 teaspoons onion powder

2 teaspoons all-natural sea salt

2 teaspoons freshly ground black pepper

4 cups frozen peas

4 cups Mashed Potatoes and Cauliflower (see recipe in Chapter 15)

Flavorful Turkey Breast

Turkey has long been considered the healthier alternative to other meats because of its lower saturated fat content. Spices, not fat, make for tasty turkey meat. So forget about using the "juices" of beef's fat to marinate and tenderize—instead, use turkey and baste and marinate with spices instead. With turkey, you don't sacrifice flavor for health.

1. Preheat oven to 350°F and spray a 9" x 13" dish with olive oil spray.

2. In a mixing bowl, combine the browned ground turkey breast, half of the minced onion, 2 teaspoons of the garlic powder, 2 teaspoons of the onion powder, 1 teaspoon of the salt, and 1 teaspoon of the pepper, and blend well.

3. Layer the meat on the bottom of the pan, cover with the peas, and sprinkle with the remaining minced onion.

4. Stir the remaining spices into the Mashed Potatoes and Cauliflower, and spoon over the peas, spreading evenly.

5. Bake at 350°F for 30 minutes, or until mashed cauliflower begins to turn golden.

PER SERVING Calories: 149.08 | Fat: 1.26 g | Protein: 17.41 g | Sodium: 461.54 mg | Fiber: 2.19 g | Carbohydrates: 16.70 g | Sugar: 2.40 g

Balsamic Chicken with Artichokes and Fire-Roasted Tomatoes

Balsamic vinegar makes this dish slightly sweet and tangy, and brings out the best of the delicious flavors of the chicken, fire-roasted tomatoes, and artichokes.

INGREDIENTS | SERVES 2

2 boneless, skinless chicken breasts

2 roasted red peppers

4 tablespoons balsamic vinegar

1 cup artichoke hearts

1 tablespoon olive oil

1 teaspoon all-natural sea salt

1 teaspoon freshly ground black pepper

1. Prepare a large skillet with olive oil spray over medium heat.

2. Cut chicken breasts into 1" pieces, add to the skillet with the olive oil, and sauté 5 minutes.

3. Cut peppers into 1" strips, and add to chicken. Add the vinegar to the skillet, and continue sautéing for 4 minutes.

4. Add artichoke hearts and seasonings, and sauté until chicken is cooked through and juices run clear.

PER SERVING Calories: 300.16 | Fat: 10.61 g | Protein: 28.92 g | Sodium: 1381.92 mg | Fiber: 8.35 g | Carbohydrates: 23.41 g | Sugar: 8.74 g

Spinach and Mushroom Chicken

While premade, frozen "bagged" meals seem like a great dinner option, look at all of the preservatives and sodium likely in the (lengthy) ingredient list. This quick skillet meal is short on ingredients and sodium, but big on nutrition and taste!

INGREDIENTS | SERVES 2

2 boneless, skinless chicken breasts

1 tablespoon olive oil

2 cups baby portabella mushrooms

2 cups baby spinach leaves

2 teaspoons garlic powder

1 teaspoon all-natural sea salt

1 teaspoon freshly ground black pepper

The Disease-Fighting Fungus

While granting a subtle, yet unique, flavor to whatever dish they present themselves in, mushrooms make for one of the smartest health food choices possible. Acting as a major player in the fight against illnesses and disease as serious as some forms of cancer, mushrooms are packed with strong antioxidants and anti-inflammatory properties that combine to fight bad cells and prevent them from coming back. More great reasons to include mushrooms in your meals!

1. Prepare a skillet with olive oil spray over medium heat.

2. Cut chicken into 1" pieces. Pour the tablespoon of olive oil and mushrooms into the skillet and sauté for 3–4 minutes.

3. Add chicken and sauté for 5 minutes.

4. When mushrooms are softened and chicken is thoroughly cooked through, add spinach leaves and seasonings, and sauté for 1 minute or until spinach is wilted.

5. Remove from heat and serve.

PER SERVING Calories: 230.76 | Fat: 10.67 g | Protein: 27.21 g | Sodium: 1298.85 mg | Fiber: 2.31 g | Carbohydrates: 7.15 g | Sugar: 2.35 g

Thai Coconut Chicken

This beautiful recipe is as delightful to the eyes as it is to your palate. Flavorful curry powder and coconut milk pair up perfectly with tender bites of chicken that gain even more delicious flavor from the tangy scallions and onions, sweet agave nectar, and refreshing bits of tomato.

INGREDIENTS | SERVES 2

2 boneless, skinless chicken breasts

1 teaspoon all-natural sea salt

1 tablespoon minced garlic

½ yellow onion, chopped

2 tablespoons curry powder

1 cup diced tomatoes

2 cups coconut milk

1 tablespoon agave nectar

2 tablespoons chopped scallions

Home-Cooked Thai Food

When was the last time you enjoyed a Thai dish that made you feel great after you ate it? More than likely, it tasted yummy but sat like a stone in your stomach. Skip most restaurants' poor ingredients, heavy sauces, high fat and calorie content, and possible use of MSG. Rethink Thai food as something you can make with fresh ingredients in your own kitchen!

1. Cut chicken breasts into small pieces (about ½"), and season with salt.

2. Prepare a large skillet over medium heat with olive oil spray.

3. Add garlic and onion to the skillet and sauté for 2–3 minutes.

4. Add the chicken and curry powder to the onions and sauté for 5–7 minutes.

5. Add tomatoes, coconut milk, and agave to the skillet and continue to simmer for 5 minutes, or until sauce thickens.

6. Remove from heat, plate, and garnish with chopped scallions.

PER SERVING Calories: 656.09 | Fat: 52.35 g | Protein: 30.38 g | Sodium: 1303.79 mg | Fiber: 2.81 g | Carbohydrates: 24.76 g | Sugar: 12.66 g

Chicken and Broccoli Fettuccine

A staple at buffets, chicken, broccoli, and ziti is a great flavor combination. The nutritional problem arises when you consider its heavy cream sauce and calorie-empty white pasta. Light and satisfying, this cleaned-up version will leave you energized, not feeling weighed down!

INGREDIENTS | SERVES 2

2 tablespoons olive oil

1 boneless, skinless chicken breast

1 teaspoon minced garlic

1 cup broccoli florets

2 tablespoons filtered water

1½ cups cooked whole wheat fettuccine

1 teaspoon all-natural sea salt

1. Prepare a skillet with 1 tablespoon of olive oil over medium heat.

2. Cut chicken breast into 1" pieces, and sauté for 2–3 minutes.

3. Add minced garlic, broccoli, and 1 tablespoon of water to skillet and continue sautéing for 4–5 minutes.

4. Add water as needed to prevent sticking and promote steaming.

5. Remove from heat when broccoli is slightly softened and the chicken is cooked through with juices running clear.

6. Toss the chicken and broccoli with the fettuccine and remaining tablespoon of olive oil. Season with the teaspoon of salt to taste.

PER SERVING Calories: 369.46 | Fat: 16.38 g | Protein: 19.44 g | Sodium: 1239.02 mg | Fiber: 3.10 g | Carbohydrates: 35.89 g | Sugar: 1.38 g

Pork Loin with Baked Apples

Rather than dipping your pork in applesauce, why not build apples into the meal itself? Aromatic, tasty, and satisfying, this delicious combination of salty pork and sweet baked apples will surely become one of your family's favorites!

INGREDIENTS | SERVES 4

¼ cup unsweetened applesauce

2 tablespoons filtered water

3 Gala apples, cored, peeled, and cut into slices

1 teaspoon cinnamon

1 pound pork tenderloin

1 teaspoon all-natural sea salt

1 tablespoon agave nectar

Homemade Olive Oil Spray

Rather than purchasing a canned aerosol olive oil spray, you can easily make your own at home. Just purchase a BPA-free plastic spray bottle (available at most grocery and hardware stores), and fill it with extra-virgin olive oil for a homemade, aerosol-free spray without chemicals or additives!

1. Preheat oven to 400°F and spray a 9" x 13" pan with olive oil spray.

2. Mix applesauce, water, and apples in a mixing bowl with cinnamon.

3. Layer the apples evenly in the pan, and cook for 20 minutes, or until slightly softened.

4. Place pork tenderloin in the middle of the pan and surround with apples.

5. Sprinkle the tenderloin with the sea salt, and drizzle the agave nectar over the pork and the apples.

6. Return the pan to the oven for another 30 minutes, or until the internal temperature reads 165°F.

PER SERVING Calories: 203.95 | Fat: 2.61 g | Protein: 23.85 g | Sodium: 649.6 mg | Fiber: 2.05 g | Carbohydrates: 21.95 g | Sugar: 18.0 g

Creamy Lemon Chicken

Living clean doesn't mean you have to ditch the cream . . . creaminess, that is! By using protein-rich Greek-style yogurt in place of heavy cream (which is high in fat and calories), this chicken dances in a lemon-cream sauce that will tempt your taste buds and satisfy your appetite!

INGREDIENTS | SERVES 2

2 boneless, skinless chicken breasts
½ cup freshly squeezed lemon juice
¼ cup plain Greek-style yogurt
2 teaspoons all-natural sea salt
1 teaspoon freshly ground black pepper
1 tablespoon chopped basil leaves

Be Smart about Substitutes

If you find yourself looking for something creamy but clean for dinner, don't fret. Eating clean means that you carefully select your ingredients and meals for optimum nutrition; not that you have to lose flavor or completely avoid an entire group of foods altogether. Try replacing cream with clean ingredients like Greek-style yogurt, nonfat yogurt, and almond milks that are thinned using the juices from the recipe's other ingredients. Tasty, health-conscious, and easy to find at your grocery store, substitutions can be just as flavorful without all the excess.

1. Cut chicken breasts into 1" pieces.

2. Prepare a skillet with olive oil spray over medium heat.

3. Pour lemon juice into skillet.

4. Once lemon juice begins to simmer, add the Greek-style yogurt and stir until the mixture becomes a sauce.

5. Add chicken, and simmer in sauce until chicken is cooked through and juices run clear.

6. Remove from heat and share the chicken evenly between two plates.

7. Cover chicken with lemon cream sauce, season with salt and pepper, and garnish with chopped basil.

PER SERVING Calories: 167.44 | Fat: 3.67 g | Protein: 27.64 g | Sodium: 2471.98 mg | Fiber: 0.55 g | Carbohydrates: 5.95 g | Sugar: 2.71 g

Spice-Rubbed Roasted Turkey Breast

Turkey breast gets a bad reputation for being bland. Yet it's protein-packed and can be made as flavorful as you want. This spice-rubbed recipe combines an abundance of tasty spices that infuse the turkey breast for a flavor sensation that will blow away that bad bland rep.

INGREDIENTS | SERVES 8

1 5-pound turkey breast

2 teaspoons garlic powder

2 teaspoons onion powder

1 teaspoon cayenne

1 teaspoon all-natural sea salt

1 teaspoon freshly ground black pepper

1 tablespoon olive oil

1 lemon, sliced

1. Preheat oven to 325°F, and prepare a roasting pan with olive oil spray. Set the turkey breast in roasting pan (make sure it is thawed).

2. Combine all spices in a small mixing bowl, and mix well.

3. Coat the turkey breast with the olive oil, and sprinkle spice mixture over the turkey breast. Top with lemon slices.

4. Cook the turkey breast for 1½–2½ hours, or until internal temperature reads 165–170°F.

PER SERVING Calories: 331.38 | Fat: 3.57 g | Protein: 69.11 g | Sodium: 432.97 mg | Fiber: 0.28 g | Carbohydrates: 1.26 g | Sugar: 0.08 g

Spinach-Stuffed Chicken

This indulgent combination of spinach and goat cheese stuffed in delicious chicken breasts makes for a mouthwatering (yet healthy!) meal. Packed with protein, complex carbohydrates, and plentiful vitamins and nutrients, savor every bite of this scrumptious meal for your health!

INGREDIENTS | SERVES 2

2 boneless, skinless chicken breasts

¾ cup crumbled goat cheese

1 cup baby spinach leaves, measured then chopped

1 teaspoon freshly ground black pepper

1. Preheat oven to 350°F and prepare a baking sheet with aluminum foil and olive oil spray.

2. Slice a 2"–3" pocket in each chicken breast by gliding a knife through the side, leaving the top intact to hold the stuffing in place.

3. In a mixing bowl, combine the goat cheese and chopped spinach, stuff the chicken breasts with even amounts of the mixture, and close sides securely with toothpicks.

4. Season chicken breasts with pepper and cook for 25–30 minutes or until chicken is golden brown and juices run clear.

PER SERVING Calories: 519.13 | Fat: 33.43 g | Protein: 50.14 g | Sodium: 389.20 mg | Fiber: 0.61 g | Carbohydrates: 3.06 g | Sugar: 1.89 g

Mango Chicken with Bowties

Sweet mangoes complement the healthy sautéed chicken beautifully, and the flavor is kicked up a notch by the addition of red pepper flakes. Sweet and slightly spicy, this chicken dish is a great satisfying go-to meal for any night of the week.

INGREDIENTS | SERVES 2

2 boneless, skinless chicken breasts

2 tablespoons olive oil

1 teaspoon all-natural sea salt

½ teaspoon red pepper flakes

2 mangoes, peeled and chopped into ¼" bite-sized pieces

2 cups cooked 100% whole wheat bowtie pasta

1. Prepare a large skillet with olive oil spray over medium heat.

2. Cut chicken into 1" pieces, and sauté with one tablespoon of olive oil for 4 minutes.

3. Season with the sea salt and red pepper, and add the mangoes to the skillet.

4. Continue cooking for 4–5 minutes, or until chicken is cooked through.

5. Remove chicken and mangoes from heat and toss with the bowties and remaining tablespoon of olive oil.

PER SERVING Calories: 609.78 | Fat: 18.89 g | Protein: 33.19 g | Sodium: 1271.07 mg | Fiber: 6.36 g | Carbohydrates: 78.64 g | Sugar: 31.47 g

Grilled Pesto Steak

Pesto is a great sauce for meat as well as pasta! Try this easy-to-cook steak topped with the fresh and aromatic Peppy Pesto.

INGREDIENTS | SERVES 4

2 cups Peppy Pesto (see recipe in Chapter 4)

1½ pounds flank steak

The Power of Beef

Packed with tons of natural flavor, protein is packed into every delicious bite of organic, lean meats. You can eat more than two-thirds of your daily recommended intake for protein with just four ounces of lean beef. If you take into consideration the amount of vitamins and minerals like B6, B12, iron, and zinc that accompany that whopping amount of protein, this small serving of meat is worth its weight in gold!

1. Place the flank steak in a large resealable plastic bag, and pour 1 cup of Peppy Pesto over the steak. Toss to coat, and marinate in the refrigerator for 4 hours.

2. Prepare a grill with olive oil spray over medium heat.

3. Set steak on the grill and cook for 8–10 minutes.

4. Turn the steak, cover with remaining cup of the Peppy Pesto, and continue cooking for 8–10 minutes or until internal temperature reads 160°F.

5. Remove from heat, set on a platter, and slice.

PER SERVING Calories: 615.07 | Fat: 45.64 g | Protein: 43.12 g | Sodium: 762.72 mg | Fiber: 0 g | Carbohydrates: 3.73 g | Sugar: 0 g

Spicy Beef Stir-Fry

Rather than ordering Chinese takeout that's made with who-knows-what quality of ingredients, save money and reap amazing health benefits by creating beef stir-fry at home. Juicy flank steak, a bevy of crisp vegetables, and spicy red pepper flakes will satisfy your craving for takeout!

INGREDIENTS | SERVES 4

1 tablespoon olive oil

1 cup broccoli florets

1 yellow onion, quartered

1 cup snow peas

1 cup white mushrooms

2 tablespoons minced garlic

4 tablespoons filtered water

1 pound flank steak, sliced

2 teaspoons red pepper flakes

1 teaspoon all-natural sea salt

Takeout Specialty, Specialized

There's nothing worse than ordering take-out, waiting, paying, and then being dissatisfied with the quality, ingredients, or taste. The best part about creating delicious takeout-style meals at home is that you can control everything from the ingredients, flavorings, portion sizes, side dishes, and taste. In less time than it would take to place a takeout order, you can have a healthy version of your favorite dish on your table.

1. Prepare a large skillet with 1 tablespoon of olive oil over medium heat.

2. Sauté the broccoli, onion, snow peas, mushrooms, and garlic with 2 tablespoons water.

3. Cover skillet and cook veggies for 3 minutes. Uncover, and continue cooking and tossing vegetables for 3 minutes.

4. Add the sliced steak and red pepper flakes to the skillet, adding remaining water as needed to prevent sticking and promote steaming.

5. Cook steak and vegetables until the steak is completely cooked through.

6. Sprinkle with teaspoon of salt, remove from heat, and enjoy!

PER SERVING Calories: 241.78 | Fat: 11.78 g | Protein: 26.07 g | Sodium: 661.54 mg | Fiber: 1.97 g | Carbohydrates: 7.74 g | Sugar: 2.66 g

Mmmmeatballs

Almost everyone loves meatballs—and this clean recipe won't disappoint. Alone, or paired with pasta and sauce, these meatballs will be a favorite with the whole family!

INGREDIENTS | MAKES 24 MEATBALLS; SERVING SIZE 1 MEATBALL

1 teaspoon olive oil

1 yellow onion, minced

½ red pepper, minced

½ green pepper, minced

2 teaspoons minced garlic

1 pound organic lean ground beef

1 teaspoon all-natural sea salt

1 teaspoon freshly ground black pepper

1 egg

2 slices sprouted grain bread, processed to crumbs

1. Prepare a skillet with olive oil spray over medium heat.

2. Pour olive oil in skillet and add minced onion, peppers, and minced garlic until soft. Remove from heat and allow to cool.

3. In a mixing bowl, combine ground beef, sautéed onion and peppers, salt, pepper, egg, and breadcrumbs.

4. Form mixture into 24 ping pong–sized balls.

5. Bake on an olive oil–prepared drip pan placed over a "catch pan" at 350°F for 10 minutes, turn, and continue baking for 10 minutes, or until completely cooked through.

PER SERVING Calories: 37.15 | Fat: 1.40 g | Protein: 4.48 g | Sodium: 127.88 mg | Fiber: 0.16 g | Carbohydrates: 1.40 g | Sugar: 0.28 g

Turkey Tetrazzini

This is a deliciously clean twist on the traditional recipe. Consider this recipe if you have leftover turkey from another dish!

INGREDIENTS | SERVES 6

1 cup white button mushrooms, chopped

1 cup unsweetened almond milk

1 pound cooked turkey breast, torn

2 cups cooked 100% whole wheat pasta

1 cup plain nonfat yogurt

1 cup sweet peas

1 cup crumbled goat cheese

2 teaspoons garlic powder

2 teaspoons onion powder

2 teaspoons freshly ground black pepper

1 teaspoon all-natural sea salt

1. Heat a sauté pan over medium heat. Add the mushrooms and ½ cup of the almond milk, and sauté until mushrooms are softened.

2. Preheat oven to 350°F and prepare a casserole dish with olive oil spray.

3. In a mixing bowl, combine the turkey, pasta, sautéed mushrooms, remaining almond milk, yogurt, peas, goat cheese, and spices.

4. Pour mixture into casserole dish, and bake for 30 minutes.

PER SERVING Calories: 404.51 | Fat: 15.78 g | Protein: 40.11 g | Sodium: 613.44 mg | Fiber: 2.75 g | Carbohydrates: 22.73 g | Sugar: 4.65 g

Lemon-Basil Chicken

Boring chicken breasts get a complete makeover with this recipe. Perky spices and fresh lemon slices make this dish a tasty treat that stays juicy and moist.

INGREDIENTS | SERVES 2

2 boneless, skinless chicken breasts

1 lemon, juiced

1 teaspoon all-natural sea salt

1 teaspoon garlic powder

2 teaspoons Italian seasoning

4 tablespoons chopped fresh basil leaves

1 lemon, sliced

Chicken for Versatile, Clean Protein

Brimming with protein and important B vitamins, chicken can be prepared in an astounding number of ways—so don't let it get boring! Whether it's grilled, broiled, blackened, roasted, sautéed, or baked, you can dress up this lean meat with spices, sauces, and serve it with pasta, rice, vegetables, or even fruit. The possibilities are endless, and the health benefits are astounding!

1. Preheat oven to 350°F, and prepare a 9" x 9" casserole dish with olive oil spray.

2. Place chicken breasts in the casserole dish and pour lemon juice over the breasts.

3. Sprinkle the breasts with salt, garlic powder, Italian seasoning, and basil leaves.

4. Cover the seasoned breasts with the lemon slices, and cook for 20–25 minutes, or until cooked thoroughly and juices run clear.

PER SERVING Calories: 155.95 | Fat: 3.67 g | Protein: 24.99 g | Sodium: 1267.34 mg | Fiber: 1.84 g | Carbohydrates: 6.56 g | Sugar: 1.5 g

Steak Pinwheels

Rolled in a beautiful pinwheel presentation, your eyes will appreciate this feast as much as your stomach!

INGREDIENTS | SERVES 4

2 pounds flank steak

2 teaspoons freshly ground black pepper

2 teaspoons garlic powder

1 cup baby spinach leaves, chopped

1 cup crumbled goat cheese

1 teaspoon all-natural sea salt

Iron with a Side of Iron

Most of the world's population suffers from some form of iron deficiency, and certain foods can resolve the issue. Great-tasting lean beef makes for a delicious serving of iron, and paired with iron-rich spinach, you've got one tasty way to fulfill those iron requirements. With an entrée of just 4 ounces of lean beef and 1 cup of spinach, you can fulfill more than half of your daily iron needs in just one sitting.

1. Pound flank steak to ¼" thickness, and sprinkle with 1 teaspoon of pepper and 1 teaspoon of garlic powder.

2. From one end to the middle of the flank steak (lengthwise), arrange the spinach and goat cheese.

3. Begin tightly rolling the flank steak and including as much spinach and goat cheese in each roll as possible. Continue rolling and tucking the spinach mixture until you reach the end.

4. Secure the roll with toothpicks, and set in the refrigerator for 4 hours to allow flavors to marry.

5. Preheat oven to 350°F and set up a pan below a grate prepared with olive oil spray. Sprinkle salt, pepper, and garlic powder over the steak, and set the steak on the grate. Cook for 30 minutes, or until internal temperature reaches 155–160°F.

6. Remove from heat, and slice the steak through all layers, and the shape of pinwheels will result.

PER SERVING Calories: 609.40 | Fat: 36.07 g | Protein: 65.19 g | Sodium: 911.40 mg | Fiber: 0.57 g | Carbohydrates: 3.20 g | Sugar: 1.29 g

Citrus Chicken Kebobs

Delectable citrus fruit gets skewered and squished between juicy pieces of chicken breast and makes for a unique flavor combination you're sure to enjoy. Packed with abundant nutrition, this meal doesn't lack in taste or flavor . . . it embodies it!

INGREDIENTS | SERVES 2

2 boneless, skinless chicken breasts
2 grapefruits
1 pineapple

1. Cut chicken breasts into ½" thick squares.

2. Remove the grapefruit rind and set aside the chunks. Remove the top and outside of the pineapple, and cut into ¼" squares.

3. Prepare a grill to medium heat with olive oil spray.

4. On four skewers, stack the chicken, pineapple, and grapefruit pieces (in that order) until all ingredients are skewered. Lay skewers on hot grill surface.

5. Turn frequently, and remove when chicken is completely cooked through or about 10 minutes.

PER SERVING Calories: 308.17 | Fat: 0.80 g | Protein: 4.06 g | Sodium: 4.53 mg | Fiber: 9.15 g | Carbohydrates: 80.05 g | Sugar: 62.44 g

Turkey Medallions in Mushroom Gravy

Pairing light and flavorful homemade mushroom gravy with thick slices of healthy turkey tenderloin makes for a hearty and filling meal. This recipe is a great way to make use of leftover gravy after a holiday meal.

INGREDIENTS | SERVES 4

1 turkey tenderloin, 2–3 pounds
1 teaspoon all-natural sea salt
1 teaspoon freshly ground black pepper
1 teaspoon garlic powder
4 cups cooked 100% whole wheat pasta ribbons
4 cups Mega Mushroom Gravy (see recipe in Chapter 15)

1. Preheat oven to 400°F and prepare a baking dish with olive oil spray.

2. Place the tenderloin in the baking dish, and sprinkle with the sea salt, pepper, and garlic powder. Place the tenderloin in the oven, and cook for 30–45 minutes, or until the internal temperature reaches 165°F.

3. Remove the tenderloin from the oven and allow to rest for 15 minutes. Slice the tenderloin into 1" medallions.

4. On four dishes, place a cup of the cooked pasta. Place the turkey medallions over the pasta, and top with the Mega Mushroom Gravy.

PER SERVING Calories: 629.12 | Fat: 6.19 g | Protein: 70.08 g | Sodium: 2112.66 mg | Fiber: 9.80 g | Carbohydrates: 73.71 g | Sugar: 1.62 g

Chicken Mozzarella

While the traditional chicken parmesan recipes are tasty, they're often packed with fat, calories, and sodium. By ditching the poor ingredients (most of which are found in the breading), you can enjoy this favorite Italian dish without the guilt . . . or the bloat!

INGREDIENTS | SERVES 4

4 boneless, skinless chicken breasts

1 teaspoon olive oil

4 teaspoons Italian seasoning

1 cup Tasty Tomato Sauce (see recipe in Chapter 4)

4 slices fresh buffalo mozzarella

2 tablespoons chopped basil leaves

1. Preheat oven to 350°F, and prepare a 9" x 13" casserole dish with olive oil spray.

2. Place chicken breasts in the dish, drizzle with olive oil, and sprinkle Italian seasoning over top.

3. Bake chicken for 20 minutes, remove from oven, top each breast with ¼ cup of the tomato sauce, and top with mozzarella slices and basil leaves.

4. Return to oven for 10 minutes, or until cheese is melted and chicken is cooked through with juices running clear.

PER SERVING Calories: 243.23 | Fat: 11.03 g | Protein: 31.09 g | Sodium: 584.92 mg | Fiber: 0.94 g | Carbohydrates: 3.95 g | Sugar: 2.99 g

Sweet and Spicy Pork Loin

You don't need a dozen ingredients to make a tasty meal. In fact, sometimes the most flavorful dishes are actually the simplest! That's the story behind this clean pork recipe.

INGREDIENTS | SERVES 4

1 pork tenderloin, about 1½ pounds
1 tablespoon agave nectar
2 teaspoons red pepper flakes

Surprise Your Taste Buds with Sweetness

A recipe such as this one may make pork one of your new go-to dishes. Preparing the pork with simple ingredients that create a sweet, yet spicy, flavor combination can be a welcome surprise to taste buds that have experienced only salty or savory varieties.

1. Preheat oven to 400°F, and prepare a baking dish with olive oil spray.

2. Lay the tenderloin in the center, drizzle with the agave nectar, and sprinkle the red pepper flakes over the entire loin.

3. Cook for 25–35 minutes, or until internal temperature reads 165°F.

PER SERVING Calories: 110.47 | Fat: 1.98 g | Protein: 17.72 g | Sodium: 45.0 mg | Fiber: 0.25 g | Carbohydrates: 4.87 g | Sugar: 4.41 g

Pulled Pork Sandwiches

Many people love barbecue pulled pork sandwiches, but most recipes load the pork with salt and sugar. Instead, prepare the pork in a healthier way, using healthier ingredients. Try these at your next casual get-together and enjoy the rave reviews!

INGREDIENTS | SERVES 6

1 pork tenderloin, about 1½ pounds
¼ cup filtered water
2 teaspoons all-natural sea salt
4 teaspoons garlic powder
4 teaspoons onion powder
6 100% whole wheat hamburger buns

1. Place the pork tenderloin in a slow cooker, pour the water over top, and cover.

2. Set on low setting for 8 hours. Tear pork apart every couple of hours.

3. After 8 hours, completely pull pork apart and season with the salt, garlic powder, and onion powder.

4. Prepare hamburger buns, spoon pulled pork onto each bun, and serve immediately.

PER SERVING Calories: 205.45 | Fat: 2.89 g | Protein: 16.02 g | Sodium: 1158.64 mg | Fiber: 1.60 g | Carbohydrates: 27.88 g | Sugar: 2.30 g

Citrus Chicken

The juicy citrus fruits in this recipe infuse their delicious flavors to the chicken breasts so they're moist, tender, and delectably delicious! This meal is perfect for a fresh summer dinner.

INGREDIENTS | SERVES 2

2 boneless, skinless chicken breasts
1 cup freshly squeezed orange juice
1 teaspoon all-natural sea salt
½ cup chopped pineapple
½ cup grapefruit pieces
1 lemon, sliced

1. Marinate chicken breasts in orange juice for 2 hours.

2. Preheat oven to 350°F and prepare a 9" x 9" casserole dish with olive oil spray.

3. Place chicken breasts in casserole dish, sprinkle with the sea salt, top with chopped pineapple and grapefruit pieces, and place lemon slices on top.

4. Cook for 25–30 minutes or until chicken is fully cooked through and juices run clear.

PER SERVING Calories: 241.72 | Fat: 3.79 g | Protein: 25.71 g | Sodium: 1268.61 mg | Fiber: 2.40 g | Carbohydrates: 27.13 g | Sugar: 19.15 g

Roasted Chipotle Chicken Breasts

Sliced deli meat will never be the same once you've tasted your very own chicken breast creation! Satisfying sandwiches, delicious dinners, or simple snacks can all be whipped up with this delicious chicken breast that's amazingly tasty and very versatile.

INGREDIENTS | SERVES 2

2 boneless, skinless chicken breasts
1 tablespoon olive oil
1 teaspoon all-natural sea salt
1 teaspoon freshly ground black pepper
4 chipotle peppers, minced
2 teaspoons garlic powder
2 teaspoons onion powder

1. Preheat oven to 375°F, and prepare roasting pan with olive oil spray. Set the thawed chicken breasts in the roasting pan.

2. Coat the chicken breasts with the olive oil, sprinkle with the salt, pepper, garlic, and onion powders, and top with the minced chipotle peppers.

3. Cook the chicken breasts for 30–45 minutes, or until internal temperature reads 165–170°F.

PER SERVING Calories: 219.27 | Fat: 10.376 g | Protein: 29.722 g | Sodium: 134.424 mg | Fiber: 0 g | Carbohydrates: 2 g | Sugar: 0 g

Sensational Marinated Steak

Using a lean cut of meat, softened fresh mushrooms, and sweet and tart balsamic vinegar for tenderizing, this steak recipe is one you'll happily (and healthfully) serve up anytime the craving for red meat strikes!

INGREDIENTS | SERVES 4

2 pounds London broil

1 onion, sliced

2 tablespoons minced garlic

4 tablespoons balsamic vinegar

1 tablespoon freshly ground black pepper

1 cup sliced portabella mushrooms

Mushrooms Can Ease Water Retention

Many vegetables do double duty by adding important vitamins and minerals to a dish. Mushrooms not only add important nutrients, they act as a natural diuretic as well. Naturally absorbing water, these delicious morsels provide the added benefit of slimming you down by eliminating excess water in the body. So, if you're feeling bloated or a little water-heavy, include mushrooms in your meal for taste and relief.

1. In a gallon-sized resealable plastic bag, marinate the steak, onions, garlic, vinegar, and pepper in a refrigerator for 4 hours.

2. Preheat oven to 350°F, and prepare a 9" x 13" casserole dish with olive oil spray.

3. Place the steak in the center of the casserole dish, pour marinade and onions over top, and scatter sliced mushrooms all around in the marinade.

4. Basting with marinade every 5 minutes, cook for 25–30 minutes, or until internal temperature reads 160°F.

PER SERVING Calories: 342.57 | Fat: 9.34 g | Protein: 52.60 g | Sodium: 144.76 mg | Fiber: 1.26 g | Carbohydrates: 8.56 g | Sugar: 4.14 g

Sweet Maple Roasted Turkey Breast

Turkey breast can be a blank canvas for a wide variety of flavors. By marinating the breast, pouring sweet maple syrup over the top, and basting throughout the cooking process, you can create a sweet and succulent version of your favorite healthy meat in no time!

INGREDIENTS | SERVES 8

1 5-pound turkey breast
1 tablespoon olive oil
1 cup organic maple syrup
1 teaspoon all-natural sea salt

1. Place the thawed turkey breast in a large resealable plastic bag, pour the olive oil and ½ cup of the maple syrup in the bag, toss to coat, and refrigerate for 4 hours.

2. Preheat oven to 325°F, and prepare a roasting pan with olive oil spray. Set the marinated turkey breast in the roasting pan.

3. Coat the turkey breast with the remaining maple syrup and sprinkle with the sea salt.

4. Cook the turkey breast for 1½–2½ hours, or until internal temperature reads 165–170°F.

PER SERVING Calories: 430.77 | Fat: 3.588 g | Protein: 68.88 g | Sodium: 435.579 mg | Fiber: 0 g | Carbohydrates: 27.004 g | Sugar: 23.957 g

Sensational Seafood

Tasty Tuna

This amazing tuna recipe takes the sweet taste of ginger and blends it beautifully with the crisp combination of rice wine vinegar, garlic, soy sauce, and scallions. Served alongside a beautiful sautéed vegetable medley or atop a bed of baby greens, this is a sure-to-be favorite!

INGREDIENTS | SERVES 2

2 tablespoons rice wine vinegar

2 tablespoons sliced ginger, chopped

2 tablespoons minced garlic

2 tablespoons chopped scallions

1 tablespoon low-sodium soy sauce

2 pounds tuna steaks

1 tablespoon canola oil

Marinating for Optimum Flavor

Chicken and beef aren't the only meats that benefit from marinating. By soaking cuts of fish in a heavenly combination of flavors, you can make your dish tasty on the inside and out. Simple and easy, all that's needed is an extra cup, or two, of the same sauces or spices you'll be using to cook the fish. Set the fish in a bowl or baggie with the marinade, and toss to coat, turning every 10–15 minutes. When you're ready to cook, the flavor you're hoping to bring out will already be in there!

1. In a mixing bowl, combine vinegar, ginger, garlic, scallions, and soy sauce, and mix well. Reserve 2 tablespoons of marinade and set aside. Add tuna steaks to marinade, and refrigerate 15 minutes.

2. Flip tuna steaks, and marinate another 15 minutes.

3. Prepare a large skillet over medium heat, and heat the tablespoon of canola oil.

4. Place tuna steaks in heated skillet and leave untouched for 5–6 minutes, or until the steaks are lightly browned.

5. Flip the tuna steaks and continue cooking for another 4–5 minutes, or until the steaks are lightly browned on both sides.

6. Remove from heat, plate the tuna steaks, and cover each steak with 1 tablespoon of the reserved marinade.

PER SERVING Calories: 725 | Fat: 29.114 g | Protein: 105.069 g | Sodium: 177.348 mg | Fiber: 0.783 g | Carbohydrates: 4.167 g | Sugar: 0.48 g

Coconut Shrimp

If you're ordering this seafood favorite at a restaurant, who knows how they made it or what they made it with. This simple recipe is a delicious and clean version of the delectable coconut shrimp we all know and love . . . and since you made it, you know what's in it!

INGREDIENTS | SERVES 2

1 cup vanilla almond milk

1 cup unsweetened coconut flakes

1 tablespoon canola oil

8 large shrimp, peeled and deveined

2 teaspoons agave nectar

1. In two shallow bowls, set up a dipping station with the almond milk in one dish and the coconut flakes in the other.

2. Prepare a skillet over medium heat with the 1 tablespoon of oil.

3. Submerge the shrimp in the almond milk.

4. Take shrimp, one at a time, out of the almond milk and roll in the coconut flakes to cover.

5. Place the shrimp in the skillet and cook for 2–3 minutes. Flip the shrimp, and continue cooking until the shrimp is cooked through and the coconut flakes are golden brown.

PER SERVING Calories: 248.732 | Fat: 20.624 g | Protein: 6.228 g | Sodium: 43.802 mg | Fiber: 3.614 g | Carbohydrates: 12.13 g | Sugar: 8.292 g

Mussels Marinara

Mussels don't necessarily pop to mind when you think about easy seafood dishes, but this recipe may just change your mind. Bursting with flavor from the mussels and homemade tomato sauce, this Italian favorite is just as good in its clean version!

INGREDIENTS | SERVES 2

1 tablespoon olive oil

1 teaspoon garlic, minced

2 cups Tasty Tomato Sauce (see recipe in Chapter 4)

2 teaspoons Italian seasoning

½ teaspoon red pepper flakes

1 pound mussels, cleaned and debearded

2 cups cooked 100% whole wheat linguine

Preparing Mussels with Perfect Technique

When selecting mussels, make sure they're fresh and smell of saltwater, not fish. Before cooking, check that all mussels are securely closed. Whether you're steaming, boiling, or baking them, watch to see that all of the mussels open during the cooking process and have had enough time to cook thoroughly. Toss any that have not opened. By themselves, topped with sauce, or mixed in with delicious ingredients, these tasty morsels of the sea burst with a unique flavor that makes every bite delicious.

1. Bring a large skillet to medium-high heat and add olive oil and minced garlic. Sauté 1–2 minutes, stirring constantly.

2. Add the tomato sauce and seasonings to the skillet and simmer 2–3 minutes.

3. Add the cleaned mussels to the skillet, toss, and cover the skillet for 5 minutes.

4. Once mussels are opened and sauce is simmering, remove from heat and toss with cooked linguine.

PER SERVING Calories: 535.825 | Fat: 13.594 g | Protein: 38.153 g | Sodium: 1926.348 mg | Fiber: 6.345 g | Carbohydrates: 65.369 g | Sugar: 11.256 g

Fabulous Fish Tacos

This dish is big on taste and low in fat and calories! This delightful combination of spicy fish, fresh veggies, and cool yogurt wrapped up in a whole wheat tortilla makes for a light and satisfying meal. As a bonus, it's easy to make for a dinner alone or a big family gathering.

INGREDIENTS | SERVES 2

2 tilapia fillets (about 1 pound)
1 tablespoon lime juice
1 teaspoon salt
2 teaspoons freshly ground black pepper
1 teaspoon cayenne pepper
2 100% whole wheat tortillas
2 tablespoons plain nonfat yogurt
1 tablespoon chopped cilantro
1 cup shredded romaine hearts
1 beefsteak tomato, chopped

Clean, Low-Fat Seafood

When choosing lean meats that will add protein and important vitamins and minerals to your diet, you'll be pleased with the option of delicious fish. Making for a quick meal that's packed with protein, low in saturated fat, and rich in omega fatty acids, fish is a great meal option for the health-focused individual who still values taste and great food.

1. Prepare a skillet over medium heat with olive oil spray.

2. Place tilapia fillets in the skillet, pour the lime juice over top, and season with the salt, pepper, and cayenne.

3. Cook fillets for 2–3 minutes, flip, and continue cooking until fish is cooked through and flaky.

4. Remove fillets from heat, and place on a platter.

5. Lay the tortillas flat and spread 1 tablespoon of the yogurt down each one, then sprinkle the chopped cilantro atop the yogurt.

6. Cut fillets into strips or chunks, and place on top of the cilantro and yogurt.

7. Top with shredded lettuce and chopped tomato, wrap tightly, and enjoy!

PER SERVING Calories: 126.37 | Fat: 3.241 | Protein: 4.199 | Sodium: 1383.122 mg | Fiber: 2.981 g | Carbohydrates: 21.204 g | Sugar: 3.296 g

Garlic Ginger Shrimp

The sweet and savory flavors of ginger and garlic make for a flavor explosion in this mouthwatering meal. Soaking up all the flavor of the delicious ingredients, tender shrimp make for the perfect star of this quick meal.

INGREDIENTS | SERVES 2

1 pound of medium shrimp, peeled and deveined

1 tablespoon olive oil

2 tablespoons minced garlic

2 tablespoons ginger, peeled and minced

1 cup chopped scallions

2 tablespoons filtered water

1 teaspoon all-natural sea salt

Low-Calorie Seafood Snack Options

Whether you steam and serve them cold, sauté them with your favorite flavors and serve them atop grains or pasta, chop them up in a refreshing creamy sauce, or bake them in a favorite casserole, shrimp make for a low-calorie meat option. With a light taste that takes flavor from other ingredients, shrimp are versatile, healthy, and packed with vitamins and minerals.

1. Combine the shrimp, olive oil, garlic, ginger, and ½ cup of scallions in bowl, and marinate for 1 hour.

2. Prepare a skillet over medium heat with olive oil spray.

3. Pour shrimp mixture into the hot skillet and sauté for 4–5 minutes.

4. Add water as needed to prevent sticking and promote steaming.

5. When shrimp is pink and cooked through, remove from heat, split between two plates, and garnish with remaining ½ cup of scallions and sprinkle with salt.

PER SERVING Calories: 341.473 | Fat: 11.215 g | Protein: 46.993 g | Sodium: 1521.361 mg | Fiber: 1.717 g | Carbohydrates: 11.426 g | Sugar: 2.644 g

Citrus Fish with Jalapeño Yogurt

The sweet bite of citrus fruit marinates and permeates the delicious grouper fillets in this recipe. Paired with cool, yet spicy, creamy yogurt, this fish dish will keep your taste buds singing!

INGREDIENTS | SERVES 2

2 grouper fillets (about 1 pound)

1 teaspoon freshly grated lime zest

½ cup chopped pineapple

½ cup chopped grapefruit

1 clementine, peeled and separated

2 tablespoons freshly squeezed lemon juice

3 tablespoons plain nonfat yogurt

1 jalapeño pepper, seeds removed and minced finely

1 teaspoon agave nectar

1. Preheat oven to 350°F and spray a 9" x 13" baking dish with olive oil spray.

2. Lay fillets in the baking dish and sprinkle with the lime zest. Cover the fillets with the pineapple, grapefruit, clementine pieces, and drizzle the lemon juice over the fillets.

3. Bake fish for 25 minutes or until cooked through and flaky.

4. In a small mixing bowl, combine yogurt, minced jalapeño, and agave.

5. Remove fish from oven, and serve with the yogurt as a dipping sauce.

PER SERVING Calories: 305.843 | Fat: 3.305 g | Protein: 45.575 g | Sodium: 133.111 mg | Fiber: 3.046 g | Carbohydrates: 23.11 g | Sugar: 18.75 g

Sesame-Seared Tuna

One of the tastiest ways to eat tuna is sushi-style! Delicious and nutritious, the natural flavors of great quality tuna are heightened in this recipe with the addition of ginger, rice wine vinegar, and shallots. Seared, and served rare, good quality tuna is a must for this dish!

INGREDIENTS | SERVES 2

½ cup rice wine vinegar

½ cup sesame oil

2 tablespoons agave nectar

2 tablespoons freshly grated ginger

2 tablespoons minced shallots

1 tablespoon minced garlic

2 tuna steaks (about 1 pound)

½ cup sesame seeds

¼ cup chopped scallions

1 tablespoon olive oil

1. Combine vinegar, sesame oil, agave, ginger, shallots, and garlic in a large dish. Reserve half of the marinade. Set the tuna steaks in the other half of the marinade in a dish for 1 hour, turning after 30 minutes to allow both sides to soak completely.

2. Pour the sesame seeds in a shallow dish, and dip steaks into the sesame seeds to cover completely.

3. Heat the olive oil in a skillet to medium heat, and place the tuna steaks in the oil.

4. Sear the tuna steaks for 30 seconds to 1 minute on each side.

5. Remove steaks from heat, garnish with chopped scallions, plate, and serve the reserved marinade as a dipping sauce.

PER SERVING Calories: 1104.917 | Fat: 90.416 g | Protein: 59.771 g | Sodium: 96.906 mg | Fiber: 5.228 g | Carbohydrates: 16.039 g | Sugar: 0.928 g

Spicy Chipotle Grilled Shrimp

This is a delicious shrimp dish with a kick supplied by the spicy chipotle peppers. Try it alone or atop a mound of brown rice or shredded lettuce. Light and satisfying, this is a great meal for lunch, dinner, or anytime a craving for spiciness hits!

INGREDIENTS | SERVES 4

4 chipotle peppers

½ yellow onion

1½ tablespoons olive oil

2 tablespoons cilantro

1 lime, juiced

2 pounds medium shrimp, peeled and deveined

Chipotles Maintain Great Metabolism

If you like spice and kick, you're in luck! Research from numerous studies on the effects of thermogenics on metabolism have shown that foods such as hot peppers and similar spicy additions that cause an increase in your internal temperature for even just a short period of time cause your metabolism to increase, meaning more fat and calorie burn. Low in calories, high in vitamins and minerals, and a good source of complex carbohydrates, peppers like chipotles and chilies can make for a more efficient metabolism with each delicious bite.

1. In a food processor, combine the chipotle peppers, onion, olive oil, cilantro, and the freshly squeezed juice of the lime, and process well until the mix becomes a paste-like sauce.

2. Pour the mixture into a covered dish, set the shrimp in the marinade, and toss to coat. Marinate for 1 hour or more, tossing occasionally.

3. Prepare a grill with olive oil over medium heat.

4. Skewer the shrimp onto grill-safe skewers, and place on the grill grate.

5. Grill the shrimp for 3 minutes, turn the skewers to flip the shrimp, and marinate the shrimp with a brush. Continue to turn the shrimp and brush with the marinade until cooked through.

6. Remove the shrimp skewers from the grill and serve.

PER SERVING Calories: 262.882 | Fat: 5.61 g | Protein: 45.763 g | Sodium: 33.493 mg | Fiber: 0.703 g | Carbohydrates: 5.088 g | Sugar: 0.866 g

Baked Tilapia with Peppers and Onions

Baked fish can get a little boring . . . if you don't spice it up just right. The delicious flavor combination of peppers and onions infuse this fish dish with a light but powerful taste that will definitely change your idea of ho-hum baked fish.

INGREDIENTS | SERVES 2

2 tilapia fillets (about 1 pound)
2 teaspoons garlic powder
2 teaspoons freshly ground black pepper
1 teaspoon all-natural sea salt
1 yellow onion, sliced
½ red pepper, sliced
½ yellow pepper, sliced
1 green pepper, sliced
2 tablespoons freshly squeezed lemon juice

1. Preheat oven to 350°F, and prepare a 9" x 13" glass baking dish with olive oil spray.

2. Set the tilapia fillets in the dish and sprinkle with the garlic powder, black pepper, and salt.

3. Cover the fillets with the onions and peppers, and drizzle the lemon juice over top.

4. Bake at 30–35 minutes, or until entire fillet is flaky and cooked through.

PER SERVING Calories: 51.811 | Fat: 0.29 g | Protein: 1.875 g | Sodium: 1188.695 mg | Fiber: 2.825 g | Carbohydrates: 12.305 g | Sugar: 4.208 g

Sweet and Spicy Salmon

This salmon is sweetened up with the amazing flavor of agave, and spiced up with the hot bite of red pepper flakes. Talk about a versatile dish that is heart-healthy, brain-healthy, and absolutely mouthwatering!

INGREDIENTS | SERVES 2

3 tablespoons agave nectar
2 tablespoons red pepper flakes
2 salmon fillets (about 1 pound)
1 teaspoon all-natural sea salt
½ teaspoon cayenne pepper

Salmon's Health Benefits

Although salmon is most famous for being omega-rich, the benefits don't stop there. Just 4 ounces also provides a clean source of more than half of your daily requirement of protein, more than 100 percent of your daily need for vitamin D, and more than half of the important B vitamins.

1. Preheat oven to 350°F and spray a 9" x 13" baking dish with olive oil spray.

2. In a mixing bowl, combine the agave and red pepper flakes.

3. Set the fillets in the baking dish and sprinkle with the salt and cayenne pepper.

4. Generously spoon the agave and red pepper mixture over the fillets, and bake for 25 minutes, or until flaky.

PER SERVING Calories: 336.339 | Fat: 15.193 g | Protein: 45.131 g | Sodium: 1279.172 mg | Fiber: 1.562 g | Carbohydrates: 3.252 g | Sugar: 0.594 g

Creamy Dill Salmon

A creamy combination of yogurt and dill top the salmon in this unique recipe.

INGREDIENTS | SERVES 2

¼ cup plain low-fat Greek-style yogurt
3 tablespoons dried dill
2 teaspoons garlic powder
2 teaspoons all-natural sea salt, divided
2 salmon fillets (about 1 pound)

1. Preheat oven to 350°F, and prepare a 9" x 13" glass baking dish with olive oil spray.

2. In a small mixing bowl, combine yogurt, dill, garlic powder, and 1 teaspoon of salt.

3. Set fillets in the baking dish and sprinkle with a teaspoon of salt. Spoon the dill yogurt over the fillets.

4. Bake for 25–30 minutes, or until fillets are flaky and completely cooked through.

PER SERVING Calories: 327.707 | Fat: 14.231 g | Protein: 44.934 g | Sodium: 2458.527 mg | Fiber: 0.27 g | Carbohydrates: 2.095 g | Sugar: 0.068 g

Shrimp Kebobs

Kebobs aren't just for chicken and steak. This delectable recipe makes a satisfying plate of juicy shrimp and crisp vegetables grilled over a flame and seasoned just perfectly. You can't go wrong with all of these fresh ingredients!

INGREDIENTS | SERVES 2

1 pound large shrimp, peeled and deveined
1 Vidalia onion, cut into 1" pieces
1 green pepper, cut into 1"pieces
1 red pepper, cut into 1" pieces
1 yellow pepper, cut into 1" pieces
1 tablespoon olive oil
2 teaspoons garlic powder
1 teaspoon all-natural sea salt
1 teaspoon freshly ground black pepper

1. Heat a grill to medium heat, and prepare skewers.

2. Skewer the shrimp and vegetables in alternating order.

3. Paint the skewered shrimp and veggies lightly with the tablespoon of olive oil, and sprinkle with the spices.

4. Grill for 2–3 minutes on each side, or until shrimp is pink and completely cooked through.

PER SERVING Calories: 366.798 | Fat: 11.039 g | Protein: 48.215 g | Sodium: 1520.249 mg | Fiber: 4.504 g | Carbohydrates: 18.186 g | Sugar: 6.691 g

Shrimp Scampi

The original recipe for this dish uses a lot of butter, oil, and sodium. This cleaned-up version keeps the delicious flavors that make this meal so scrumptious, while cutting out the ingredients that make it not-so-hot in the health or waistline areas.

INGREDIENTS | SERVES 2

1 tablespoon olive oil

1 shallot, minced

1 tablespoon minced garlic

1 teaspoon all-natural sea salt

1 teaspoon red pepper flakes

2 teaspoons Italian seasoning

1 lemon, juiced

1 pound large shrimp, peeled and deveined

1 lemon, ½ juiced and ½ sliced

2 cups cooked 100% whole wheat fettuccine

1. Heat a large skillet over medium heat, and drizzle 1 tablespoon oil in pan.

2. Sauté shallot, minced garlic, salt, red pepper, and Italian seasoning in the juice of 1 lemon until shallot is translucent.

3. Add shrimp to skillet and sauté until pink and in the shape of a "c." Squeeze the juice of ½ of the remaining lemon over the shrimp and steam for 1 more minute.

4. Remove shrimp from heat, toss with cooked whole wheat pasta, and garnish with thin slices of the remaining ½ lemon. Add salt to taste.

PER SERVING Calories: 1149.907 | Fat: 14.312 g | Protein: 75.559 | Sodium: 1525.842 | Fiber: 8.716 g | Carbohydrates: 175.259 g | Sugar: 7.202 g

Flaky Fish with Quinoa and Red Onions

While many people refrain from cooking types of fish, many white fish like snapper, tilapia, grouper, and cod offer up a wide variety of health benefits as well as a blank canvas for many flavors.

INGREDIENTS | SERVES 2

1 cup dry organic quinoa

2 cups filtered water

½ tablespoon garlic powder

½ tablespoon onion powder

1 pound snapper

½ red onion, chopped

1 tablespoon extra-virgin olive oil

1 teaspoon all-natural sea salt

Quinoa for Balanced Nutrition

Because quinoa is actually a seed related to deep green leafy vegetables, this uncommon food is rich in complex carbohydrates. Add to the complex carbohydrates the rich protein source quinoa also provides, and you've got a completely balanced nutritious food that combines two of the most necessary dietary components in one!

1. Rinse the quinoa thoroughly, and combine with the water in a medium saucepan over medium heat, and bring to a boil. Reduce heat to low, add half of the garlic powder and onion powder, and simmer for 15 minutes.

2. Preheat oven to 400, and prepare a 9" x 13" glass baking dish with olive oil spray.

3. Place the snapper fillets in the baking dish and cover with the chopped red onions. Drizzle with the olive oil and sprinkle with the garlic and onion powders. Bake for 25–30 minutes or until fish is cooked through and flaky.

4. Remove the quinoa from the heat, transfer to a separate dish, and fluff with a fork.

5. Transfer the fish and onions to the quinoa dish, flake with a fork, and toss to combine. Sprinkle with salt to taste.

PER SERVING Calories: 620.303 | Fat: 14.972 g | Protein: 58.774 g | Sodium: 1330.253 mg | Fiber: 6.869 g | Carbohydrates: 59.997 g | Sugar: 1.331 g

Feisty Fish Tabbouleh

For years, bodybuilders and fitness competitors have been using these protein-packed fillets to stay trim, lean, and free of excess fat and water. Tilapia fillets will fill you up lightly without weighing you down.

INGREDIENTS | SERVES 2

½ onion, minced

½ red pepper, chopped

1 tablespoon olive oil

2 tilapia fillets (about 1 pound)

1 teaspoon cumin

1 teaspoon all-natural sea salt

½ teaspoon cayenne pepper

1 tablespoon filtered water

2 cups cooked bulgur

Try Bulgur!

Bulgur is a great grain that can be used as a substitute for heavy pasta or potatoes. You can find it, organic or not, in the rice and pasta aisle of your local grocer. While you can also find it premade, try making the homemade variety to suit your exact taste . . . plus, you'll know what's in it!

1. In a skillet over medium heat, sauté the onion and red pepper for 3–5 minutes in the olive oil. Season fish fillets with cumin, salt, and cayenne and add fish fillets to skillet.

2. Add 1 tablespoon water to prevent sticking and promote steaming, and cook fish fillets for 5 minutes and flip.

3. Continue cooking fish for 5 minutes, or until fish is completely cooked through and flaky.

4. Flake fish apart, and thoroughly combine with onion and pepper.

5. Add fish, onion, and pepper to cooked bulgur, mix well, and serve.

PER SERVING Calories: 267 | Fat: 13.24 g | Protein: 19.161 g | Sodium: 1254 mg | Fiber: 4.37 g | Carbohydrates: 20.41 | Sugar: 1.188 g

Sweet Scallops with Chives

Lots of people don't make scallops at home because they assume that they're difficult to prepare. Try this recipe to set the record straight! It's simple to make but has restaurant-quality taste!

INGREDIENTS | SERVES 2

2 tablespoons agave nectar
1 tablespoon coconut milk
1 pound bay scallops
2 tablespoons fresh chopped chives
1 teaspoon all-natural sea salt

Health Benefits of Scallops

Packed with vitamin B$_{12}$, omega-3s, and manganese, scallops make for great cardiovascular guardians that promote optimum blood flow, prevent clots, and help maintain low blood pressure.

1. In a small dish, combine the agave and coconut milk, and soak the scallops for 1 hour.

2. Preheat oven to 400°F and prepare a 9" x 9" glass baking dish with olive oil spray.

3. Set the scallops in the prepared baking dish. Pour the coconut milk mixture over the scallops and top with the chopped chives and sea salt.

4. Bake for 20–30 minutes, or until scallops are firm.

PER SERVING Calories: 305 | Fat: 1.528 g | Protein: 48.283 g | Sodium: 1772 mg | Fiber: 0.1 g | Carbohydrates: 11.87 g | Sugar: 11.55 g

Mexican Fish

Always perfect together, hearty black beans, sweet corn, cool tomatoes, and mildly peppery poblanos and onion need no more than simple salt and pepper to highlight their flavors and make every bite better than the last! Try it served over rice, by itself, or wrapped in a tortilla.

INGREDIENTS | SERVES 2

1 tablespoon olive oil
½ cup soaked black beans
½ cup kernel corn
½ cup chopped tomatoes
½ cup chopped poblano peppers
½ cup yellow onion, chopped
2 tilapia fillets (about 1 pound)
1 teaspoon all-natural sea salt
1 teaspoon freshly ground black pepper

1. Preheat oven to 350°F, and prepare a 9" x 9" baking dish with olive oil spray.

2. In a mixing bowl, combine the olive oil, beans, corn, tomatoes, peppers, and onion.

3. Place fillets in the baking dish, sprinkle with the salt and pepper, and cover with the olive oil and bean mixture.

4. Bake for 25–30 minutes, or until cooked through and flaky.

PER SERVING Calories: 185.15 | Fat: 7.647 g | Protein: 5.842 g | Sodium: 1375.48 mg | Fiber: 6.392 g | Carbohydrates: 26.141 g | Sugar: 6.506 g

Shrimp Salad

This is a delicious spin on the traditional shrimp salad. Contrary to the traditional recipe's mayonnaise base and few vegetables (if any), this recipe contains a light and refreshing blend of yogurt, celery, onion, and amazing spices!

INGREDIENTS | SERVES 2

1 pound cooked and chilled large shrimp, shells removed

½ cup chopped celery

¼ cup minced onion

½ cup plain nonfat yogurt

1 teaspoon garlic powder

1 teaspoon onion powder

1 teaspoon all-natural sea salt

1 teaspoon freshly ground black pepper

1. Chop shrimp into bite-sized pieces.

2. Combine shrimp, celery, onion, yogurt, and spices in a covered dish.

3. Refrigerate shrimp salad for 1 hour to allow flavors to marinate. Serve chilled.

PER SERVING Calories: 298.878 | Fat: 5.994 g | Protein: 48.515 g | Sodium: 1565.533 mg | Fiber: 1.403 g | Carbohydrates: 10.271 | Sugar: 4.368 g

Shrimp Salad for Any (Healthy!) Mealtime

Light recipes that utilize fresh ingredients with healthy benefits are great any time, so why limit delicious varieties to only one mealtime? Simple recipes like this Shrimp Salad can be used as a delicious dinner entrée, a light lunch, a quick snack, or even an appealing appetizer. Just remember to enjoy what you eat and eat what you enjoy!

Mediterranean Fish Bake

This dish blends hearty ingredients that carry their own unique flavors: roasted red peppers, artichokes, olives, and (of course) snapper. Seasoned with spices that bring out the natural aromas and taste of the fish, this is one recipe you're sure to enjoy time and again.

INGREDIENTS | SERVES 2

1 tablespoon olive oil
½ cup sliced black olives
½ cup roughly chopped artichoke hearts
1 roasted red pepper, cut in strips
½ yellow onion, chopped
2 plum tomatoes, chopped
2 snapper fillets (about 1 pound)
1 teaspoon garlic powder
1 teaspoon freshly ground black pepper
1 teaspoon all-natural sea salt

1. Preheat oven to 350°F and prepare a 9" x 9" glass baking dish with olive oil spray.

2. In a small mixing bowl, combine olive oil, olives, artichokes, roasted red pepper, onion, and tomatoes and combine well.

3. Place fillets in the baking dish and sprinkle with the garlic powder, pepper, and sea salt.

4. Cover the fillets with the mix. Bake for 25–30 minutes, or until fish is cooked through and flaky.

PER SERVING Calories: 445.54 | Fat: 17.376 g | Protein: 52.033 | Sodium: 1681.836 mg | Fiber: 11.75 g | Carbohydrates: 26.526 g | Sugar: 6.022 g

Mediterranean Means Flavorful

With each and every ingredient of Mediterranean dishes strategically used for flavor, there's not a single addition that doesn't serve a purpose. In addition to taste, though, you'd be surprised how much each ingredient contributes to the healthier functioning of the body and the brain. Rich in fish and healthy oils, natural ingredients, and creative ways to promote flavors like fire-roasting, the Mediterranean diet is one that is well-known for food combining for optimum health. Follow suit and enjoy!

Tuna Noodle Casserole

Can't decide what's for dinner? Fall back on this American favorite. The clean version uses healthy whole wheat pasta, calcium-rich almond milk, and fresh mushrooms.

INGREDIENTS | SERVES 4

2 cans solid white albacore tuna, drained

1½ cups unsweetened almond milk, divided

1½ cups plain nonfat yogurt, divided

1 cup minced mushrooms

1 teaspoon all-natural sea salt

1 teaspoon freshly ground black pepper

1 teaspoon garlic powder

1 teaspoon onion powder

2 cups cooked 100% whole wheat pasta ribbons

1 cup crumbled goat cheese

1. In a mixing bowl, combine the tuna, 1 cup of almond milk, 1 cup yogurt, mushrooms, and seasonings. Blend ingredients well, and fold in pasta.

2. Preheat oven to 350°F, and prepare a casserole dish with olive oil spray.

3. Pour the tuna mixture into the casserole dish and top with the crumbled goat cheese.

4. Bake for 30–45 minutes or until hot and bubbly.

PER SERVING Calories: 586.098 | Fat: 27.838 g | Protein: 48.747 g | Sodium: 1158.524 mg | Fiber: 5.642 | Carbohydrates: 32.695 g | Sugar: 2.42 g

Shrimp Casserole

With a light, tasty food that's naturally low in fat and calories and as versatile as shrimp, why not utilize it in as many dishes as you can? This is an easy one-pot meal that the whole family will enjoy.

INGREDIENTS | SERVES 8

1 pound cooked shrimp, shells removed

1 cup plain nonfat yogurt

½ cup plain low-fat Greek-style yogurt

½ cup water chestnuts, chopped

1 cup chopped scallions

1½ cups crumbled goat cheese

2 teaspoons garlic powder

1 teaspoon all-natural sea salt

2 teaspoons freshly ground black pepper

2 cups cooked brown rice

1. Preheat oven to 350°F and prepare a 9" x 13" casserole dish with olive oil spray.

2. In a mixing bowl, combine shrimp, yogurts, water chestnuts, scallions, half of the goat cheese, and seasonings. Fold in rice and mix thoroughly.

3. Pour the shrimp mixture into the prepared baking dish, and sprinkle remaining goat cheese over top.

4. Cook for 30–45 minutes.

PER SERVING Calories: 475.698 | Fat: 18.706 g | Protein: 30.131 g | Sodium: 552.355 mg | Fiber: 2/769 g | Carbohydrates: 45.778 g | Sugar: 4.031 g

Lemon Fish with Capers and Cream

One of the best parts of clean eating is that you can replicate poor food choices so you don't have to avoid some of your favorite meals. That's what this recipe is all about—making a light cream sauce rather than a heavy, fat-laden cream one.

INGREDIENTS | SERVES 2

2 tilapia fillets (about 1 pound)
1 tablespoon olive oil
1 teaspoon all-natural sea salt
1 teaspoon freshly ground black pepper
½ cup freshly squeezed lemon juice
½ cup plain nonfat yogurt
2 tablespoons capers, rinsed

1. In a large skillet over medium heat, place the fish fillets in the tablespoon of olive oil. Sprinkle the fillets with the salt and pepper and sauté for 4 minutes.

2. Add the lemon juice to the skillet and turn the fish, continuing to sauté for about 4 minutes, or until the fish is cooked through.

3. Remove the fillets from the skillet, place each fillet on a serving dish, and reduce the heat of the skillet to low.

4. Stir in the nonfat yogurt and capers to the remaining lemon juice, and use a wooden spoon to stir and remove cooked bits from the pan.

5. Once the sauce is combined, about 1 minute, remove from heat and pour over the fillets.

PER SERVING Calories: 247.488 | Fat: 14.053 g | Protein: 21.345 g | Sodium: 1550.668 mg | Fiber: 0.802 g | Carbohydrates: 11.915 g | Sugar: 8.356 g

Shrimp Pasta Bake

Tender shrimp, sweet peas and corn, creamy yogurt, and strong goat cheese crumbles combine in an easy one-dish casserole you can pop in the oven while you help the kids with their homework.

INGREDIENTS | SERVES 8–10

1 pound of large cooked shrimp, shells removed

2 cups cooked 100% whole wheat rotini pasta

2 shallots, sautéed

2 teaspoons minced garlic

2 cups nonfat yogurt

1 cup sweet peas

1 cup corn kernels

1 teaspoon all-natural sea salt

1 teaspoon freshly ground black pepper

1 teaspoon onion powder

½ cup crumbled goat cheese

1. Preheat oven to 350°F, and prepare a casserole dish with olive oil spray.

2. In a mixing bowl, combine shrimp, pasta, sautéed shallots, garlic, yogurt, peas, corn, and salt, pepper, and onion powder. Blend thoroughly.

3. Pour the mixture into the casserole dish, and top with the crumbled goat cheese.

4. Bake for 30–45 minutes or until cooked through.

PER SERVING Calories: 369.44 | Fat: 9.463 g | Protein: 23.093 g | Sodium: 458.496 mg | Fiber: 3.428 g | Carbohydrates: 47.919 g | Sugar: 4.988 g

All Kinds of Good-For-You Carbs

Packing any meal with delicious and nutritious ingredients makes for a great meal, but loading up on complex carbohydrates can work wonders on the stomach, body, and mind. Fueling up with clean carbohydrates like fresh vegetables and whole grain pastas, you can be sure that your body has clean fuel that it can burn efficiently. The vitamins and minerals that are intact in fresh veggies (and stripped otherwise) make for sweet, spicy, or salty additions that can take the flavor in any direction imaginable. Carbo-loading is a great way to prepare for a big day or a grueling workout, so choose wisely, choose smart, choose complex carbs.

CHAPTER 8

Very Vegetarian

Vegetarian Meatloaf

Vegetarian cuisine can be as modern or classic as you desire. This traditional meal gets a complete makeover, using delicious vegetables and rice for a vegetarian version of meatloaf. It's so packed with flavor your family might not even notice that it's missing the meat!

INGREDIENTS | SERVES 4

1 cup cooked brown rice

1 pound portabella mushrooms, minced and sautéed

1 small yellow onion, minced

1 red pepper, minced

1 cup spinach, chopped

1 cup wheat germ, plain

2 eggs, beaten

1 tablespoon Worcestershire sauce

2 teaspoons garlic powder

2 teaspoons onion powder

2 teaspoons all-natural sea salt

2 teaspoons freshly ground black pepper

1. Preheat oven to 350°F and prepare a 9" x 9" baking dish with olive oil spray.

2. Combine all ingredients in a mixing dish, and refrigerate for 1 hour.

3. Pour mix into the center of the baking dish and form into a loaf.

4. Bake at 350°F for 30–45 minutes or until cooked through.

PER SERVING Calories: 251.79 | Fat: 6.24 g | Protein: 14.53 g | Sodium: 1280 mg | Fiber: 7.85 g | Carbohydrates: 38.56 g | Sugar: 5.45

Hearty Ingredients for Filling Substance

If you need to thicken up any dishes, you can easily choose from a couple of clean ingredients. Brown rice is a great filler that you can add to vegetarian meat-like recipes to give a similar texture. Beans are another great thickening agent that can be added to soups, and thick yogurts like Greek-style varieties can be very helpful in thickening up smoothies, soups, sauces, and such.

Veggie Lasagna

This recipe uses whole wheat pasta, fresh vegetables, homemade tomato sauce, and buffalo mozzarella for mouthwatering taste and health benefits without any guilt.

INGREDIENTS | SERVES 12

1 package of 100% whole wheat lasagna noodles

1 tablespoon olive oil

1 small zucchini, sliced thinly

1 green pepper, diced

3 teaspoons minced garlic

1 yellow onion, minced

1 pound portabella mushrooms, sliced

6 cups of prepared Tasty Tomato Sauce (see recipe in Chapter 4)

4 teaspoons Italian seasoning, divided

2 eggs

1 cup cottage cheese

1 cup plain Greek-style yogurt

12 thin slices of fresh buffalo mozzarella

Ditch the Processed Cheese

The clean lifestyle makes a major point of still eating things you love, but trying to use fresh ingredients and healthier alternatives whenever possible. Cheese is one thing that's common in the standard American diet that really shouldn't be. Heavily processed, fat-packed, calorie-laden, dairy cheeses like deli slices and prepackaged singles are terribly unnatural. Fresh buffalo mozzarella and crumbled goat cheese are two natural alternatives that are very versatile, minimally processed, and taste great. These are two healthy options you can live with.

1. Preheat oven to 350°F and prepare a 9" x 13" baking dish with olive oil spray.

2. Prepare a large pot with water over medium-high heat. Cook noodles until al dente, remove, rinse, and cool.

3. Prepare the rinsed noodle pot with one tablespoon olive oil, and add the zucchini, pepper, minced garlic, and onion. Sautee for 2–3 minutes, and add the mushrooms, sauce, and half of the Italian seasoning. Reduce heat to medium and simmer for 15 minutes.

4. Combine the eggs, cottage cheese, and yogurt in a mixing bowl.

5. Pour 1 cup of the sauce in the bottom of the dish to coat. Layer (for two layers) half of the noodles, followed by half of the sauce, dollops of the yogurt mix spread, and half of the mozzarella cheese.

6. Layer, in the same order for a second time, and sprinkle the mozzarella topping with remaining Italian seasoning.

7. Bake for 30–45 minutes, or until bubbly and cooked through.

PER SERVING Calories: 396.98 | Fat: 6.15 g | Protein: 18.19 g | Sodium: 785.4 mg | Fiber: 5.22 g | Carbohydrates: 68.09 g | Sugar: 11.22 g

Cabbage Rolls

Cabbage rolls can be a satisfying snack or delicious dinner. They do require a little extra time to cook, but they're well worth the effort. Packed with fresh veggies and lots of taste, this is one unique meal that will pleasantly surprise you.

INGREDIENTS | SERVES 12

1 tablespoon olive oil

1 red pepper, minced

1 yellow pepper, minced

½ red onion, minced

1 small zucchini, minced

3 garlic cloves, crushed and minced

12 red cabbage leaves

1 cup cooked brown rice

1 egg, beaten

1 teaspoon all-natural sea salt

1 teaspoon freshly ground black pepper

1 teaspoon Worcestershire sauce

1 cup Tasty Tomato Sauce (see recipe in Chapter 4)

Vitamins, Minerals, and Polyphenols, Oh, My!

Just one cup of delicious red cabbage goes a long way in terms of health benefits. Almost 100 percent of the daily recommended serving of vitamin K, more than half of the day's vitamin C, and a great amount of healthy fiber are all packed into just one cup of red cabbage. In addition to these great vitamins, the polyphenols (that are made up of an astounding percentage of anthocyanins) not only give red cabbage its beautiful deep red-purple coloring, but also work diligently to fight cancers by preventing free radical damage.

1. Prepare a large skillet with the tablespoon of olive oil over medium heat, and sauté the red pepper, yellow pepper, red onion, zucchini, and garlic until softened, about 5 minutes.

2. In a large pot, boil cabbage leaves for 2–4 minutes, or until soft.

3. In a mixing bowl, combine the rice, sautéed veggies, egg, salt, pepper, and Worcestershire sauce and blend well.

4. Put a ¼ cup mound of the mix in the center of each cabbage leaf, roll to close, and tuck the ends.

5. Prepare a slow cooker to low heat, and pour a couple of tablespoons of the sauce in the bottom to coat and prevent sticking. Place the rolls in the slow-cooker, and cover with sauce.

6. Cook for 8 hours, remove from heat, plate, and sprinkle with salt and pepper.

PER SERVING Calories: 67.32 | Fat: 1.88 g | Protein: 2.58 g | Sodium: 329.95 mg | Fiber: 3.12 g | Carbohydrates: 11.40 g | Sugar: 4.45 g

Stuffed Poblanos

These stuffed peppers are a feast for your eyes and a satisfying treat for your tummy. Clean, green, and not too spicy, these are a quick and easy answer to an empty party platter or the perfect at-home snack.

INGREDIENTS | SERVES 12

6 poblano peppers

1 onion, minced

1 yellow pepper, minced

1 red pepper, minced

1 jalapeño pepper, minced (remove seeds before mincing if desired)

1 cup cooked brown rice

1 teaspoon garlic powder

1 cup crumbled goat cheese

1. Cut poblanos in half lengthwise. Set all peppers on a foil-lined baking sheet prepared with olive oil spray.

2. Combine minced onion, yellow pepper, red pepper, jalapeño pepper, and cooked rice. Blend ingredients well, and season with garlic powder.

3. Spoon the mixture evenly into the poblano halves, and top with goat cheese crumbles.

4. Bake at 400°F for 20–25 minutes or until cheese is bubbly and peppers are cooked through.

PER SERVING Calories: 120.33 | Fat: 6.93 g | Protein: 6.82 g | Sodium: 67.89 mg | Fiber: 1.18 g | Carbohydrates: 8.22 g | Sugar: 2.51 g

Baked Veggie Pasta

Meat's not needed in this delicious dish. Plentiful veggies make for a beautiful—and easy to prepare—meal that will pleasantly satisfy even the pickiest of eaters. Getting your recommended vegetable servings is a breeze with this one-dish meal.

INGREDIENTS | SERVES 5

2 cups chopped spinach

3 roasted red peppers, sliced

2 cups portabella mushrooms, sliced

2 cups artichoke hearts, crushed

½ red onion, sliced

1 zucchini, sliced into ¼" rounds

2 cups black olives, sliced

2 cups crumbled goat cheese

4 cups cooked 100% whole wheat penne pasta

1. Prepare a 9" x 13" baking dish with olive oil spray, and preheat oven to 350°F.

2. In a mixing bowl, combine the spinach, red peppers, mushrooms, artichoke hearts, onion, zucchini, olives, and cheese. Fold in the pasta and combine well.

3. Pour the veggie pasta mixture into the prepared baking dish and bake for 30–45 minutes.

PER SERVING Calories: 635.96 | Fat: 33.25 g | Protein: 34.78 g | Sodium: 737.71 mg | Fiber: 13.66 g | Carbohydrates: 56.58 g | Sugar: 5.66 g

Pasta Primavera

Boring veggie pasta this is not! Fuel up for anything, anytime with this filling dish that sports rich complex carbohydrates that perfectly complement the hearty pasta.

INGREDIENTS | SERVES 4

4 tablespoons olive oil, divided

1 small zucchini, sliced

1 small yellow squash, sliced

1 yellow onion, sliced

1 large carrot, sliced

4 tablespoons filtered water (as needed)

1 cup baby portabella mushrooms, sliced

½ red pepper

1 cup broccoli florets

2 teaspoons garlic powder

2 teaspoons freshly ground black pepper

2 teaspoons all-natural sea salt

1 teaspoon onion powder

4 cups cooked 100% whole wheat rigatoni pasta

1. Prepare a skillet with 1 tablespoon of olive oil over medium heat, and sauté the zucchini, squash, onion, and carrots for about 7 minutes, adding water when needed to prevent sticking and promote steaming.

2. Add mushrooms, red pepper, and broccoli, and continue to sauté for another 7 minutes, or until all vegetables are slightly softened.

3. Pour the prepared pasta into a mixing bowl and add veggies and seasonings. Drizzle remaining 2–3 tablespoons of olive oil (for desired taste) over the pasta and toss to coat.

PER SERVING Calories: 457.05 | Fat: 15.65 g | Protein: 14.49 g | Sodium: 1216.04 mg | Fiber: 13.22 g | Carbohydrates: 71.86 g | Sugar: 7.28 g

Mushroom and Asparagus Bake

All it takes are two types of veggies to give this dish all the clean flavor it needs. Kids like bowtie pasta shapes so much, they may not even notice they're eating the veggies, too!

INGREDIENTS | SERVES 8

2 cups chopped asparagus spears

1 cup portabella mushrooms, sliced

1 cup oyster mushrooms, sliced

1 cup cremini mushrooms, sliced

1 tablespoon olive oil

1 tablespoon filtered water

4 cups 100% whole wheat farfalle pasta

2 teaspoons garlic powder

1 teaspoon freshly ground black pepper

1 cup plain nonfat yogurt

1 cup plain Greek-style yogurt

1 cup crumbled goat cheese

Low-Sodium Benefits and Diuretic Veggies

By combining fresh vegetables (like mushrooms and asparagus that are well-known for being natural diuretics) with a low-sodium meal that supplies rounded nutrition, everyone wins.

1. Preheat oven to 350°F, and prepare a 9" x 13" baking dish with olive oil spray.

2. Prepare a skillet with olive oil spray over medium heat. Sauté the asparagus and mushrooms in the olive oil until slightly softened, about 4–6 minutes, adding water as needed to prevent sticking and promote steaming.

3. Remove veggies from heat and toss with the pasta in a mixing bowl. Add the seasonings, yogurts, and goat cheese, and blend thoroughly.

4. Pour the mix into the baking dish and bake for 30 minutes, or until cooked through and bubbly.

PER SERVING Calories: 336.19 | Fat: 14.09 g | Protein: 18.55 g | Sodium: 140.24 mg | Fiber: 6.11 g | Carbohydrates: 37.13 g | Sugar: 6.20 g

Very Veggie Casserole

The amount and variety of vegetables in this casserole are reason enough to indulge in this fabulous dish. Filling your home with a delicious aroma—and satisfying your cravings for a hearty casserole dish—this recipe will become a go-to favorite.

INGREDIENTS | SERVES 4

1 cup sweet peas

1 cup kernel corn

1 cup sautéed sliced mushrooms

1 cup carrot, cut into matchsticks

½ cup yellow onion, minced

1 cup plain nonfat yogurt

1 cup plain Greek-style yogurt

1 tablespoon garlic powder

1 tablespoon onion powder

2 teaspoons freshly ground black pepper

4 cups cooked 100% whole wheat farfalle pasta

½ cup crumbled goat cheese

1. Preheat oven to 350°F and prepare a 9" x 13" baking dish with olive oil spray.

2. In a mixing bowl, combine the vegetables and yogurts with the seasonings.

3. Fold in the cooked pasta and pour into the prepared baking dish, and top with the crumbled goat cheese.

4. Bake for 30 minutes, or until cooked through and bubbly.

PER SERVING Calories: 587.91 | Fat: 16.23 g | Protein: 28.97 g | Sodium: 187.13 mg | Fiber: 14.62 g | Carbohydrates: 89.05 g | Sugar: 14.91 g

Tofu Spaghetti

Everyone loves spaghetti. Since tofu soaks up the flavors of the foods around it, your family will get its health benefits while enjoying this Italian feast.

INGREDIENTS | SERVES 4

1 tablespoon olive oil

1 package extra firm tofu, crumbled

2 cups Tasty Tomato Sauce (see recipe in Chapter 4)

4 cups cooked 100% whole wheat spaghetti

2 teaspoons all-natural sea salt

4 slices fresh buffalo mozzarella

¼ cup chopped basil

1. In a large skillet over medium heat, combine the olive oil and crumbled tofu and sauté until slightly browned.

2. Add the spaghetti sauce to the sautéed tofu and bring to a simmer.

3. Remove the tofu and sauce from the heat and move to a large serving bowl and thoroughly combine with the pasta and salt.

4. Plate, and garnish with the mozzarella slices and chopped basil.

PER SERVING Calories: 375.13 | Fat: 10.31 g | Protein: 18.72 g | Sodium: 1940.38 mg | Fiber: 4.48 g | Carbohydrates: 52.19 g | Sugar: 7.21 g

Italian Portabella Burgers

This delicious recipe takes the beefy taste of portabella mushrooms and gives them the Italian twist we all crave sometimes. Simple to create, this hearty sandwich is a great way to skip the beef but still enjoy the grill!

INGREDIENTS | SERVES 2

2 large portabella caps

2 tablespoons olive oil

4 teaspoons Italian seasoning

½ cup Tasty Tomato Sauce (see recipe in Chapter 4)

2 slices fresh buffalo mozzarella

Mushroom Storage for Optimal Nutrition

Did you know that where and how you store your mushrooms can affect their nutrient content? Recent studies have shown that the best way to preserve the valuable vitamins and nutrients that make mushrooms so great is to store them in a cold refrigerator set to about 38°F as soon as you get them home. Even setting them on a counter or in a pantry for a short period of time can reduce the number and quality of phytonutrients.

1. Prepare a grill with olive oil spray over medium heat.

2. Paint the tops of the portabella caps with the olive oil, then flip and paint the gills also. Season both sides of both caps with 2 teaspoons of the Italian seasoning (reserving the other 2 teaspoons).

3. Place the portabellas on the grill with the gills facing down. Cook for about 5 minutes, and flip.

4. Continue to cook the caps for about 5 more minutes. Top the gills of each cap with ¼ cup of the sauce, a slice of the mozzarella, and the remaining Italian seasoning.

5. Close the grill lid for 2–3 minutes (checking periodically), until the cheese is melted.

6. Remove from heat, and serve.

PER SERVING Calories: 194.52 | Fat: 17.03 g | Protein: 5.69 g | Sodium: 416.56 mg | Fiber: 2.01 g | Carbohydrates: 6.85 g | Sugar: 4.85 g

Tempeh Fajitas

Fajitas don't have to be packed with processed ingredients and sodium-laden spices to be absolutely delicious. This recipe combines nutritious tempeh, fresh vegetables, and health benefits galore . . . all wrapped up in filling, nutritious tortillas!

INGREDIENTS | SERVES 4

1 tablespoon olive oil

1 tablespoon freshly squeezed lime juice, divided

1 teaspoon cayenne pepper, divided

1 container tempeh, cut into bite-sized pieces

1 yellow onion, sliced

1 green pepper, sliced

1 red pepper, sliced

4 tablespoons plain nonfat yogurt

4 100% whole wheat tortillas

1 tablespoon chopped green chili peppers

Tempeh: The New Tofu

When you're having a craving for some meatless dishes that will satisfy your cravings for healthy, hearty—without beans, lentils, or veggies—tempeh is an additional option to the traditional tofu. Made from fermented soybeans, tempeh has a light nutty flavor, with the same type of texture as tofu, and the wonderful appeal of taking on the flavors of whatever meal it composes. Packed with protein, B vitamins, manganese, and riboflavin, tempeh is a delicious option for meatless meals that still need a little something.

1. In a large skillet, drizzle olive oil over medium heat and add half of the lime juice, half of the cayenne, and all of the tempeh to the heated skillet. Sautee for about 5 minutes, or until lightly browned and slightly firm.

2. Toss in onions, green and red peppers, and remaining cayenne pepper. Sauté until veggies are slightly softened, but still have crunch.

3. In a small mixing bowl, combine the yogurt and remaining lime juice.

4. Drizzle the lime yogurt down the center of each tortilla.

5. Remove the tempeh and veggies from the heat, and place in the center of each tortilla.

6. Top each fajita with the chopped green chilies, and serve.

PER SERVING Calories: 260 | Fat: 12.41 g | Protein: 14.06 | Sodium: 205.29 mg | Fiber: 2.06 g | Carbohydrates: 25.78 g | Sugar: 3.34 g

Tofu Enchiladas

Enchiladas can be an absolute nightmare for a healthy diet. No more does this delicious dish have to weigh down your waistline and wear down your health, however! Loaded with the freshest ingredients, you can happily enjoy these amazing enchiladas guilt-free.

INGREDIENTS | SERVES 6

2 tablespoons olive oil

2 packages of firm tofu, crumbled

1 yellow onion, minced

1 red pepper, minced

2 tablespoons filtered water

1 cup plain nonfat yogurt

½ cup plain low-fat Greek-style yogurt

1 teaspoon all-natural sea salt

¼ cup chopped green chilies

6 100% whole wheat tortillas

1 teaspoon cayenne pepper

1. Prepare a large skillet with 1 tablespoon of olive oil over medium heat.

2. Add crumbled tofu, and sauté until slightly browned. Remove the tofu from the skillet and add the onion and red pepper to the heat with 1 tablespoon of the water. Sauté until slightly softened. Remove from heat and let cool with the cooked tofu.

3. After tofu and veggies have cooled, add yogurts, salt, and chopped green chilies, and blend well.

4. Prepare a large baking dish with olive oil spray and preheat oven to 350°F.

5. Set all tortillas out in a row, and place even amounts of the tofu mixture in the center of each.

6. Roll each tortilla's ends in first, and then roll to result in a completely enclosed enchilada.

7. Place tortillas face-down in the baking dish, paint with remaining tablespoon of olive oil, and sprinkle with cayenne pepper.

8. Bake for 30 minutes.

PER SERVING Calories: 255.33 | Fat: 11.62 g | Protein: 13.23 g | Sodium: 659.38 mg | Fiber: 1.87 g | Carbohydrates: 24.78 g | Sugar: 6.95 g

Stuffed Red Peppers

Filled with delicious ingredients that make each pepper a hearty meal in itself, this is an amazingly beautiful recipe to make for your family, or to serve to sure-to-be-awed guests.

INGREDIENTS | SERVES 4

4 red peppers, tops and ribs removed
1 tablespoon olive oil
2 teaspoons minced garlic
1 zucchini, chopped
1 yellow squash, chopped
½ red onion, chopped
2 fire-roasted red peppers, chopped
2 teaspoons onion powder
2 teaspoons freshly ground black pepper
1 teaspoon all-natural sea salt
2 cups cooked brown rice
¼ cup crumbled goat cheese

Bell Peppers: Nature's Multivitamin

Did you know that by indulging in just one cup of red bell peppers, you can satisfy a number of your daily recommendations for vitamins? One cup of bell pepper contains almost 300 percent of your vitamin C needs and more than 100 percent of your vitamin A. In addition to those important vitamins, the carotenoids that give them their beautiful flavors also pack peppers full of powerful antioxidants that help to fight off illnesses and disease.

1. In a large pot of boiling water, submerge the peppers and boil for 2–4 minutes, remove, and let cool.

2. Prepare a large sauté pan with the tablespoon of olive oil over medium heat. Add the minced garlic and chopped zucchini, squash, and onion, and sauté until slightly softened.

3. Add the roasted red pepper, onion powder, pepper, and salt, and continue to sauté until all flavors are well blended.

4. Move the vegetables from the heat to a large mixing bowl, and combine with the rice.

5. Stuff the peppers with the rice and vegetable mixture, top with the crumbled goat cheese, and bake for 20–25 minutes, or until cheese is bubbly.

PER SERVING Calories: 268.44 | Fat: 9.78 g | Protein: 9.73 g | Sodium: 651.28 mg | Fiber: 6.54 g | Carbohydrates: 38.03 g | Sugar: 7.57 g

Ultimate Black Bean Burgers

Hearty black bean burgers make for protein-packed veggie-burger alternatives that can easily be topped with your favorite clean ingredients, such as corn salsa, eggs, or the traditional crisp lettuce and juicy tomato.

INGREDIENTS | SERVES 4

2 cups black beans, soaked for 24–48 hours and drained

1 egg

2 slices sprouted grain bread

½ green bell pepper

½ red onion

2 garlic cloves

1 teaspoon onion powder

1 teaspoon cumin powder

1 teaspoon all-natural sea salt

1. In a large mixing bowl, mash black beans and egg together thoroughly.

2. In a food processor, reduce bread slices to fine crumbs, and combine crumbs with the mashed black beans.

3. Put the green bell pepper, onion, and garlic in the food processor and mince finely.

4. Mix all of the ingredients (including the spices) together in the mixing bowl, combine thoroughly, and form into patties.

5. On a grill prepared with olive oil spray over medium heat, grill patties for 5–8 minutes per side until cooked through and slightly crispy on the edges.

PER SERVING Calories: 186.28 | Fat: 2.47 g | Protein: 10.66 g | Sodium: 1092.34 mg | Fiber: 7.83 g | Carbohydrates: 30.83 | Sugar: 3.88 g

Egg-Cellent Salad

With all of the poor foods replaced with clean ones that provide great health benefits, you can eat this on toast, on a salad, or just on its own.

INGREDIENTS | SERVES 4

12 eggs, boiled and shells removed
1 cup celery, roughly chopped
½ cup scallions, chopped
2 tablespoons red wine vinegar
¼ cup plain nonfat yogurt
2 teaspoons freshly ground black pepper
1 teaspoon garlic powder

Eggs for Pregnancy Health

While eggs are a well-known source of protein, toting an amazing 5½ grams of protein per egg, these white wonders are also packed with a special vitamin, choline. Necessary for reducing inflammation, promoting circulation, reducing bad cholesterol, and maintaining a healthy weight, choline is an important part of any diet that can be satisfied with scrumptious eggs.

1. Place the eggs into a large covered dish and crush with a fork.

2. Add the celery, scallions, and red wine vinegar and fold gently to avoid making a paste.

3. Fold in the yogurt and seasonings to blend well.

4. Cover and refrigerate for 1 hour or until completely chilled through.

PER SERVING Calories: 56.35 | Fat: 3.07 g | Protein: 4.12 g | Sodium: 67.53 mg | Fiber: 0.83 g | Carbohydrates: 3.02 g | Sugar: 1.48 g

Tomato-Basil Rigatoni

Even a simple pasta-and-sauce recipe can be full of poor ingredients if you buy everything at the store. Instead, homemade tomato sauce, whole wheat pasta, and the freshest ingredients make this familiar favorite a satisfying and healthy delight.

INGREDIENTS | SERVES 2

2 cups cooked 100% whole wheat rigatoni pasta

2 cups Tasty Tomato Sauce (see recipe in Chapter 4)

1 teaspoon garlic powder

¼ cup chopped basil

2 tablespoons Italian seasoning

½ cup fresh buffalo mozzarella, crumbled

1. In a large mixing bowl, combine the hot cooked pasta with the Tangy Tomato Sauce, garlic powder, chopped basil, and Italian seasoning.

2. Plate pasta, and sprinkle the mozzarella crumbles over top.

PER SERVING Calories: 369.85 | Fat: 8.05 g | Protein: 17.96 g | Sodium: 1461.81 mg | Fiber: 6.41 g | Carbohydrates: 58.16 g | Sugar: 11.54 g

Spice It Up!

If you're looking to jazz up a dish you fear might be on the bland side, don't reach for that salt! Rather than using sodium (which is already consumed in high amounts in many diets), fresh and dried herbs can lend a lot of taste without any of the sodium. Basil, rosemary, oregano, tarragon, cumin, cilantro, turmeric, and many more can be the pleasant pairing you're looking for!

Squash Casserole

If you're looking for a hearty meal packed with delicious and fresh ingredients, look no further. This one-pot meal is perfect for a fall evening.

INGREDIENTS | SERVES 6–8

1 large zucchini
1 large yellow squash
1 butternut squash
2 tablespoons olive oil
2 tablespoons Italian seasoning
1 tablespoon paprika
2 teaspoons all-natural sea salt
2 cups cooked brown rice
½ cup crumbled goat cheese

Versatile Deliciousness

If you're looking for a wonderful fresh vegetable that can be made creamy, crunchy, sweet, or salty, look no further than summer squash. Blended with fresh ingredients, natural nectars, or light and savory seasonings, you can create the most amazing-tasting dishes. Whether you'd like a sautéed dish, a hearty casserole, or a creamy soup, summer squash is an easy, inexpensive ingredient that makes for a delicious and nutritious meal any day or night of the week.

1. Cut the squashes into bite-sized pieces (strips or rounds), of comparable size.

2. Preheat the oven to 400°F and prepare a 9" x 13" baking dish with olive oil spray.

3. In a large mixing bowl, combine the squashes, olive oil, and seasonings, and mix well.

4. Fold in the rice and goat cheese, and bake for 35–45 minutes or until cooked through and bubbly.

PER SERVING Calories: 154.37 | Fat: 8.95 g | Protein: 5.83 g | Sodium: 640.69 mg | Fiber: 1.445 g | Carbohydrates: 13.01 g | Sugar: 1.01 g

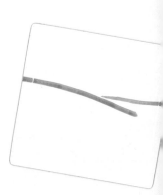

Chicken Patties

Rather than buying one of those packages of frozen chicken patties from the store, why not make your own right at home? Besides tasting better, these have much less sodium and preservatives than the storebought kind.

INGREDIENTS | SERVES 4

1 tablespoon plus 1 teaspoon olive oil

1 cup mushrooms, diced

1 yellow onion, diced

1 teaspoon minced garlic

2 slices sprouted grain bread

1 pound garbanzo beans (soaked and drained)

2 eggs

1 teaspoon all-natural sea salt

1 teaspoon freshly ground black pepper

1 teaspoon cumin

1 teaspoon curry powder

Garbanzo Beans for Extended Satisfaction

Fiber-packed garbanzo beans have long been heralded as a nutritious element of any snack or meal. Now, though, recent studies conducted in 2010 and reported in *Appetite* magazine showed that participants who consumed 104 grams of garbanzo beans daily reported a more satisfying, longer-lasting feeling of fullness along with fewer cravings, and less of an appetite for fattening and sugary foods. With all of those fabulous facts and the countless ways you can create delicious dishes using garbanzo beans, there's no reason not to enjoy these fibrous treats daily.

1. In a large sauté pan, sauté the teaspoon of olive oil, mushrooms, onions, and minced garlic until soft and cooked through. Move from the skillet to a mixing bowl, and save skillet for cooking the completed patties.

2. In a food processor, reduce the bread slices to fine crumbs and move to the mixing bowl.

3. Add the garbanzo beans, tablespoon of olive oil, and eggs to the food processor and blend well. Move to the mixing bowl.

4. Add the sautéed veggies to the crumbs and bean mix, and thoroughly combine all ingredients with the seasonings.

5. Bring the skillet back to medium heat, and spray with olive oil spray.

6. Form the mix into patties, and set into the preheated skillet. Cook for 4–6 minutes on each side, until cooked through.

PER SERVING Calories: 547.81 | Fat: 14.05 g | Protein: 27.74 g | Sodium: 758.85 mg | Fiber: 21.00 g | Carbohydrates: 81.40 g | Sugar: 14.14 g

Italian Tofu Bake

Rather than indulging in a fattening dose of chicken parmesan, try this delightful Italian tofu recipe that is delicious, light, and completely satisfying.

INGREDIENTS | SERVES 4

2 slices sprouted grain bread

3 tablespoons Italian seasoning, divided

2 eggs

1 package extra-firm tofu

2 cups Tasty Tomato Sauce (see recipe in Chapter 4)

4 slices fresh buffalo mozzarella

Tofu Instead of White Meat . . . or the Other White Meat . . . or the Other White Meat

Being a vegetarian or vegan doesn't mean you can't enjoy the same flavors found in delicious dishes that include chicken, turkey, fish, etc. Just replace the meat components of your favorite meal with tofu, prepare it in the same manner, and serve it in the same delicious delivery. You can enjoy that chicken parmesan, turkey tetrazzini, beefy burger, or whatever your heart desires.

1. In a food processor, reduce the bread slices to fine crumbs, then move the crumbs to a shallow dish and combine with 1 tablespoon of the Italian seasoning.

2. In a shallow bowl, beat the 2 eggs until frothy.

3. Slice the tofu into 8 equal slices.

4. Preheat oven to 400°F and cover a baking sheet with foil and olive oil spray.

5. Dip the tofu slices into the egg, dredge in the breadcrumbs, and place on the baking sheet. Repeat process with all of the tofu slices.

6. Bake the tofu slices for 10–15 minutes, or until golden brown and slightly crispy. Flip, and continue to bake for 8–10 minutes.

7. Remove the tofu from the oven, spoon ¼ cup of the sauce on each, and top with half of a mozzarella slice and Italian seasoning.

8. Return the tofu to the oven and continue baking until cheese is melted.

PER SERVING Calories: 242.59 | Fat: 10.93 g | Protein: 19.14 g | Sodium: 1011.47 mg | Fiber: 2.31 g | Carbohydrates: 18.12 g | Sugar: 6.93 g

Great Vegan Stroganoff

This recipe creates the classic stroganoff dish in a much lighter, healthier, and beneficial way by swapping out the poor ingredients with ones that are fresh, healthy, and provide nutrition and taste. Dive into this delicious plate of goodness without any guilt or remorse!

INGREDIENTS | SERVES 4

1 tablespoon olive oil

2 packages extra-firm tofu, crumbled

1 yellow onion, minced

1 cup sliced mushrooms

1 teaspoon garlic powder

2 tablespoons low-sodium soy sauce

12 ounce container nonfat cottage cheese

2 tablespoons plain Greek-style yogurt

16 ounces 100% whole wheat noodles, cooked

2 teaspoons freshly ground black pepper

1. Prepare a large skillet with olive oil over medium heat.

2. Sautee tofu crumbles and onion in the olive oil for 7 minutes, or until cooked through.

3. Add the mushrooms, garlic powder, and soy sauce, and combine well.

4. Stir in the cottage cheese and Greek yogurt, until the ingredients become a thick sauce. Remove from the heat.

5. In a large bowl, combine the cooked noodles, tofu mixture, and pepper, and blend well. Serve immediately.

PER SERVING Calories: 417.74 | Fat: 12.69 g | Protein: 29.33 g | Sodium: 373.95 g | Fiber: 3.17 g | Carbohydrates: 46.09 g | Sugar: 6.85 g

Portabella Cakes

Talk about hearty! This delicious recipe turns plain old portabella mushroom caps into mouthwatering greatness. All of the amazing health benefits that you get from these fresh ingredients only increase their appeal.

INGREDIENTS | SERVES 2

2 slices sprouted grain bread

2 tablespoons Italian seasoning

2 eggs

1 tablespoon olive oil

2 large portabella mushroom caps

½ cup crumbled goat cheese

1 teaspoon all-natural sea salt

1 teaspoon freshly ground black pepper

Mushrooms Substitute for Beef Patties?

Have you ever seen those gigantic portabella mushroom caps and wondered, "What do you do with those?" Well, a recipe that replaces the meat of a sandwich with these beautiful mushrooms is tasty, and astoundingly nutritious. Cutting the fat and calories from traditional beef patties can make for a healthier option with just as much flavor, if not more. So, the next time you pass by those large portabella caps, pick up a pack, and try out a delicious burger or tasty entrée with those as the star!

1. In a food processor, reduce the bread slices to crumbs, and combine with the Italian seasoning. Move to a shallow dish.

2. In a shallow dish, beat eggs thoroughly.

3. Prepare a skillet with olive oil over medium heat.

4. Submerge the caps in the egg and then dredge in the breadcrumbs.

5. Place the caps in the skillet, and cook for 5–8 minutes, or until lightly golden.

6. Flip the caps, and place the crumbled goat cheese on top of the caps.

7. Continue cooking for 5–7 minutes, remove from heat, salt and pepper to taste, and enjoy.

PER SERVING Calories: 497.97 | Fat: 32.57 g | Protein: 29.03 g | Sodium: 1658.81 mg | Fiber: 2.14 g | Carbohydrates: 23.61 g | Sugar: 4.53 g

Ratatouille

Ah, ratatouille, the forgotten dish. Clean and chock-full of fresh vegetables that give the body and mind energy and the "good" carbohydrates we all need, this is a one-pot meal you don't want to miss.

INGREDIENTS | SERVES 4

1 tablespoon olive oil
1 large eggplant, cut into 1" cubes
2 tablespoons minced garlic
1 zucchini, cut in ½" pieces
1 yellow squash, cut in ½" pieces
2 Roma tomatoes, cut in slices
1 green pepper, cut in ½" pieces
1 red pepper, cut in ½" pieces
½ cup crumbled goat cheese

Combining Vegetables for Flavor and Nutrition

When you're struggling to reach those daily vegetable servings, try whipping up a hearty dish that focuses on vegetables solely. Combining flavorful vegetables in a tomato sauce with garlic and cheese makes for a splendid dish that doesn't even taste like it consists of only vegetables. Adding extras like basil and spices only improves the flavor and nutritional content, so don't be shy.

1. Preheat oven to 350°F and coat a large casserole dish with olive oil spray.

2. In a large skillet, heat the tablespoon of olive oil over medium heat. Add the eggplant, and sauté until softened, about 10 minutes.

3. Place the eggplant on the bottom of the casserole dish for the first layer, and top with the minced garlic.

4. Layer the zucchini, followed by the squash, then the tomatoes, and the peppers last.

5. Cover the top layer with the goat cheese, and bake for 30–40 minutes.

PER SERVING Calories: 229.26 | Fat: 14.03 g | Protein: 12.17 g | Sodium: 108.65 mg | Fiber: 7.16 g | Carbohydrates: 16.96 g | Sugar: 8.42 g

Veggie Fajitas

These meatless fajitas make great use of fresh onions and peppers in a delicious blend of spices, all cooled off with cold yogurt, crisp lettuce, and tomato, wrapped in whole wheat tortillas. You won't miss the meat!

INGREDIENTS | SERVES 4

1 tablespoon olive oil
1 yellow onion, cut into thin strips
1 green bell pepper, cut into thin strips
1 red bell pepper, cut into thin strips
1 yellow bell pepper, cut into thin strips
2 teaspoons cumin powder
1 teaspoon red pepper flakes
1 teaspoon all-natural sea salt
2 tablespoons filtered water
4 100% whole wheat tortillas
½ cup plain nonfat yogurt
1 cup romaine lettuce, chopped
1 cup tomatoes, chopped

1. Prepare a large skillet with the tablespoon of olive oil over medium heat.

2. Add the onion and peppers to the skillet, and sauté until slightly softened.

3. Sprinkle the peppers and onion with the cumin, red pepper flakes, and salt. Combine, using the water as needed to promote steaming and prevent sticking.

4. Lay tortillas flat, spread yogurt down the center of each tortilla, load the onion and peppers evenly into the tortillas, and cover with the lettuce and tomato.

5. Serve immediately.

PER SERVING Calories: 186.22 | Fat: 7.30 g | Protein: 5.39 g | Sodium: 803.40 mg | Fiber: 3.93 g | Carbohydrates: 26.39 g | Sugar: 6.70 g

Eggplant, Portabella, Spinach, and Mozzarella Stacks

No need for buns here! This hearty helping of delicious veggies is its own self-contained vessel of greatness. The portabella mushroom caps make for a thick and juicy bun-like wrap for the delicious fire-roasted eggplant, wilted spinach, and melted mozzarella.

INGREDIENTS | SERVES 2

1 large eggplant, cut into ¼–½" full length slices

2 tablespoons olive oil

1 teaspoon all-natural sea salt

1 teaspoon freshly ground black pepper

4 large portabella mushrooms

1 cup baby spinach leaves

2 slices fresh buffalo mozzarella

Excellent Eggplant for Brain Food

Eggplant is not only delicious, nutritious, and extremely versatile, it contains a powerful anthocyanin (the cancer-fighting chemicals that cause the deep, vibrant colors in fruits and vegetables) called nasunin that make it a powerful brain food. Nasunin acts as a powerful protector against free radical damage (which wreaks havoc on cells, causing dangerous changes like cancer) in the brain by protecting the fats that are so important to the brain's optimal functioning and conveying of messages to the rest of the body. By enjoying eggplant, you're not only satisfying your hunger and your taste, you're doing your brain a world of good.

1. Prepare a grill with olive oil spray and bring to medium heat.

2. Paint the eggplant slices with olive oil, sprinkle with salt and pepper, and place on the grill. Grill for 8–10 minutes, or until the eggplant is cooked through.

3. Paint the portabella mushroom caps' gills with olive oil, sprinkle with salt and pepper, and place on the grill. Paint the tops, and flip to grill the tops after about 5–7 minutes.

4. Toss the spinach leaves in the remaining olive oil, and sprinkle with remaining salt and pepper.

5. While still on the heat, immediately after flipping the caps with the gills facing up, place half of the spinach on each of the two caps and 1 slice of mozzarella on each of the other two caps. Continue cooking until the spinach is wilted and the cheese is slightly melted.

6. Remove the caps from the grill, and stack the eggplant slices on the two caps with spinach. Top with the mozzarella caps, and enjoy!

PER SERVING Calories: 313.23 | Fat: 21.03 g | Protein: 13.14 g | Sodium: 1389.73 mg | Fiber: 12.11 g | Carbohydrates: 23.98 g | Sugar: 11.00 g

Very Veggie Burgers

Just like the chicken patties, you could buy veggie burgers at any supermarket. Making them at home, however, means less money spent, control of the ingredients, and control of the flavor. Try these out, and you'll never go storebought again.

INGREDIENTS | SERVES 4

2 slices sprouted grain bread

2 teaspoons garlic powder

2 teaspoons onion powder

1 pound of garbanzo beans, soaked and drained

½ red pepper, minced

½ green pepper, minced

½ zucchini, minced

¼ cup black or green olives, minced

½ red onion, minced

2 eggs

1 teaspoon all-natural sea salt

1 teaspoon freshly ground black pepper

1. In a food processor, reduce bread slices to crumbs with the garlic and onion powders, and move to a large mixing bowl.

2. Process the garbanzo beans, red pepper, green pepper, zucchini, olives, and onion until finely minced, and add to breadcrumbs.

3. Add the eggs to the mixture, and blend well. Form into even patties and sprinkle with the salt and pepper to taste.

4. Prepare a skillet over medium heat with olive oil spray, and place the patties into the skillet. Cook for 4–6 minutes on each side, or until golden brown and slightly crispy.

PER SERVING Calories: 521.89 | Fat: 11.0 g | Protein: 27.70 g | Sodium: 833.443 mg | Fiber: 21.32 g | Carbohydrates: 82.69 g | Sugar: 14.25 g

CHAPTER 9

Vegan

Tex-Mex Tacos

Sometimes you just can't resist the urge for delicious, spicy tacos. With this clean recipe, you don't have to! You won't miss the extra sodium or fat since you're using fresh peppers and onions, crumbled tofu, homemade salsa, and flavorful cumin!

INGREDIENTS | SERVES 4

1 tablespoon olive oil
1 package extra firm tofu, crumbled
1 red pepper, cut into strips
1 yellow onion, cut into strips
1 tablespoon filtered water
1 cup Scrumptious Salsa (see recipe in Chapter 4)
2 teaspoons cumin
4 100% whole wheat tortillas

1. Prepare a large skillet with olive oil spray over medium heat. Add olive oil and tofu, and sauté until lightly browned.

2. Add the pepper and onion to the skillet with the water, and sauté until the vegetables are slightly softened. Add the salsa to the skillet with the seasonings and bring to a simmer.

3. Remove from the heat, and spoon the tofu mix into the tortillas' centers.

PER SERVING Calories: 213.70 | Fat: 8.37 g | Protein: 10.02 g | Sodium: 613.39 mg | Fiber: 3.13 g | Carbohydrates: 25.87 g | Sugar: 5.53 g

Thai Tofu

Sometimes ordering out can seem like a great way to save on time. Instead, save your money and better your health with a delicious recipe like this one. Thai tofu delivers salty, spicy, and sweet all in the same delicious package. Light and scrumptious, you'll be wowed with every bite!

INGREDIENTS | SERVES 2

1 tablespoon olive oil
1 package of extra-firm tofu, crumbled
2 tablespoons minced fresh ginger
2 tablespoons minced garlic
1 tablespoon low-sodium soy sauce
1 teaspoon cayenne pepper
¼ cup chopped scallions
½ cup chopped unsalted natural cashew nuts

1. In a large skillet over medium heat, sauté the olive oil and tofu until lightly browned.

2. Add the ginger, garlic, soy sauce, and cayenne to the skillet and sauté together until cooked through. Remove from heat.

3. Plate the tofu, and garnish with the scallions and chopped cashews.

PER SERVING Calories: 501.59 | Fat: 36.25 g | Protein: 22.81 g | Sodium: 71.71 mg | Fiber: 2.99 g | Carbohydrates: 26.85 g | Sugar: 6.31 g

Bean Burritos

Once you make your own easy bean burritos, and make them exactly how you want, you'll never pick them up anywhere else but in your own kitchen. Adding jalapeño, habanero, or banana peppers can make this one spicy treat, too.

INGREDIENTS | SERVES 4

4 100% whole wheat tortillas

2 cups of Spicy Clean Refried Beans (see recipe in Chapter 4)

1 cup soaked kidney beans

2 cups cooked brown rice

2 cups plain nonfat yogurt

Bye-Bye Drive-Through

By creating delicious dishes like bean burritos and healthy hamburgers, your desire for the fast-food versions may dissipate or disappear completely. So, when you're in your kitchen experimenting, think about those foods and make 'em over.

1. Lay the tortillas on a flat surface.

2. Spread ½ cup of the refried beans down the center of each tortilla.

3. Combine the rice and kidney beans in a bowl, and put ¼ of the mixture on each tortilla.

4. Top each tortilla's rice mixture with ¼ cup of the yogurt, and wrap tightly.

PER SERVING Calories: 538.99 | Fat: 8.89 g | Protein: 26.28 g | Sodium: 793.48 mg | Fiber: 20.21 g | Carbohydrates: 89.8 g | Sugar: 7.86 g

Thai Vegetable Curry

The background of light nutty sweetness from the almond butter gives these fresh vegetables a nice flavor that's accented beautifully with the curry powder and garlic. Before you knock it, you have to try it!

INGREDIENTS | SERVES 2

1 eggplant, chopped

1 zucchini, chopped

1 tablespoon olive oil

1 cup coconut milk, divided

3 tablespoons almond butter

1 teaspoon minced garlic

1 yellow onion, minced

2 celery stalks, minced

2 teaspoons curry powder

1. In a large skillet, sauté the eggplant and zucchini in the olive oil over medium heat until softened, about 8–10 minutes.

2. Add half of the coconut milk, and all of the almond butter, minced garlic, onion, celery, and curry powder and simmer.

3. Add remaining coconut milk as a thinner if needed; remove from heat and serve hot.

PER SERVING Calories: 499.50 | Fat: 38.01 g | Protein: 9.39 g | Sodium: 65.59 mg | Fiber: 13.62 g | Carbohydrates: 40.03 g | Sugar: 19.74 g

Vegan Chili

Everybody loves chili! Well, almost everybody. The only "clean" problem with chili is that most recipes call for fatty meat as the main ingredient. Vegans rejoice . . . this recipe uses crumbled tofu as the star ingredient!

INGREDIENTS | SERVES 8

15 ounces dried black beans

15 ounces dried kidney beans

15 ounces dried garbanzo beans

15 ounces dried white beans

2 packages extra-firm tofu

1 tablespoon extra-virgin olive oil

2 cups Tasty Tomato Sauce (see recipe in Chapter 4)

2 cups chopped Roma tomatoes

2 cups fresh or frozen corn kernels

1 yellow onion, chopped

1 celery stalk, chopped

1 green pepper, chopped

4 tablespoons Italian seasoning

1 tablespoon cayenne pepper

1. Soak all bean for 24 hours, rinse, and drain.

2. In a large skillet over medium heat, sauté the crumbled tofu and olive oil until golden brown and slightly crispy.

3. In a cold slow cooker, combine all ingredients.

4. Set slow cooker to low.

5. Cook for 8–10 hours, or until ingredients are soft and flavors well-blended.

PER SERVING Calories: 708.42 | Fat: 7.22 g | Protein: 45.11 g | Sodium: 550.19 mg | Fiber: 38.17 g | Carbohydrates: 122.16 g | Sugar: 19.14 g

Garlic Ginger Tofu

Sweet ginger and garlic with a bite join forces in this recipe to deliver taste and sound nutrition. All of the clean and fresh ingredients in this tasty combination will make you wonder why you never thought to try something so simple and delicious before.

INGREDIENTS | SERVES 4

1 package extra-firm tofu
2 tablespoons agave nectar
2 tablespoons minced garlic
2 tablespoons minced ginger
2 tablespoons olive oil, divided
1 teaspoon all-natural sea salt

1. Slice the tofu into 8 equal slices.

2. Combine the agave, garlic, and ginger in a shallow dish with 1 tablespoon of the olive oil.

3. Place the sliced tofu in the mixture and refrigerate for 30 minutes, turning frequently.

4. Prepare a skillet with olive oil spray over medium heat.

5. Move the tofu slices from the marinade to the skillet, and drizzle with the olive oil and half of the marinade (reserving half for the topping).

6. Sautee the tofu slices for 10–15 minutes, or until golden brown and slightly crispy.

7. Remove the tofu from the skillet, and spoon the remaining marinade over each slice. Salt to taste.

PER SERVING Calories: 159.66 | Fat: 9.2 g | Protein: 6.34 g | Sodium: 621.83 mg | Fiber: 0.53 g | Carbohydrates: 14.06 g | Sugar: 9.9 g

Amazing Roasted Veggie Toss

*For this recipe, you'll just chop the ingredients and throw them in a dish to bake!
Besides smelling and tasting amazing, these beautiful vegetables make
for a meal full of great health benefits that will also fill you up.*

INGREDIENTS | SERVES 4

4 Idaho potatoes, washed and cut into ½" cubes

4 large carrots, cut into ½" cubes

2 yellow onions, cut into ½" chunks

2 tablespoons olive oil

1 teaspoon garlic powder

1 teaspoon onion powder

1 teaspoon turmeric

1 teaspoon Italian seasoning

Roasting for Powerful Flavor

Roasting vegetables can make for an incredibly different experience than sautéing or baking. By tossing vegetables in olive oil, roasting them in high heat, and flavoring them with delicious spices, you can create a crunchy variation of the vegetables you already know and love. Potatoes and carrots aren't the only ones great for roasting, either: Zucchini, squash, tomatoes, onions, and celery are also great options.

1. Preheat the oven to 400°F and prepare a 9" x 13" casserole dish with olive oil spray.

2. In a large resealable plastic bag, combine the potatoes, carrots, onions, olive oil, and spices, and toss to coat.

3. Pour the vegetables into the prepared baking dish.

4. Bake at 400°F for 1 hour, moving vegetables around at 30 minutes, and again at 45 minutes.

PER SERVING Calories: 285.74 | Fat: 7.22 g | Protein: 6.05 g | Sodium: 63.72 mg | Fiber: 5.99 g | Carbohydrates: 51.86 g | Sugar: 7.14 g

Roasted Vegetable and Hummus Mix-Up

This recipe takes roasted eggplant, squash, and red onion, and makes them even tastier by coating them in a homemade roasted red pepper hummus that is not only amazingly scrumptious, but can be eaten completely guilt-free.

INGREDIENTS | SERVES 4

2 tablespoons olive oil
1 eggplant, cut into ½" cubes
1 zucchini, cut into ½" cubes
1 yellow squash, cut into ½" cubes
1 red onion, into ½" slices
2 teaspoons garlic powder
1 teaspoon all-natural sea salt
2 cups Roasted Red Pepper Hummus (see recipe in Chapter 4)

Fiber Mixed with Fiber

If you're feeling like you're weighted down or slightly stopped up, dishes that combine tons of fiber may be the perfect solution. Fibrous vegetables taste even better when they're tossed in fiber-rich hummus made from the amazingly healthy and tasty garbanzo bean. Packed with loads of fiber that may do just the trick to get things moving along again, rich vegetable dishes tossed in chickpea hummus are nature's delicious solutions to modern-day issues.

1. Preheat oven to 400°F and coat a large casserole dish with olive oil spray.

2. In a large resealable plastic bag, toss the olive oil, eggplant, zucchini, squash, onion, and spices together and coat completely.

3. Pour the vegetables into the casserole dish, and cook for 1 hour.

4. Remove the vegetables, allow to cool for 10 minutes, and toss with the Roasted Red Pepper Hummus until completely coated.

5. Serve, or refrigerate in a covered dish.

PER SERVING Calories: 331.85 | Fat: 19.29 g | Protein: 12.98 g | Sodium: 1072.91 mg | Fiber: 13.78 g | Carbohydrates: 32.42 g | Sugar: 6.72 g

Sweet and Sour Tofu and Veggies

The sweet and sour sauce you'd get from your local Chinese takeout place is probably not as clean as this one. Made from all-natural ingredients, the sweetness of freshly mashed cherries combines with the salty bite of vinegar for an amazing marinade that can't be beat.

INGREDIENTS | SERVES 2

½ cup fresh cherries

1½ tablespoons vinegar

3 tablespoons agave nectar

1 scallion, minced

1 tablespoon fresh minced ginger

1 package extra-firm tofu

1. In a large bowl, mash the cherries until they are completely juiced. Discard pits, stems, and skins, and reserve juice.

2. Add the vinegar, agave, scallions, and minced ginger to the large bowl, and whisk to combine.

3. Slice the tofu lengthwise to form 8 strips, and set in the marinade for one hour.

4. Over medium heat, prepare a skillet with olive oil spray, and set the tofu in the skillet.

5. Brown both sides of the tofu for about 4–5 minutes per side.

6. Add the marinade to the skillet and bring to a simmer.

7. Remove from heat, plate tofu, and drizzle marinade over top.

PER SERVING Calories: 238.03 | Fat: 4.80 g | Protein: 12.4 g | Sodium: 63.74 mg | Fiber: 1.49 g | Carbohydrates: 38.64 g | Sugar: 33.56 g

Vegetarian Chili

Who says chili has to be loaded with fat, calories, and who-knows-how-they-made-it cheese to be satisfying and delicious. This hearty meal can serve double duty for snacks and lunches or for a delicious dinner a couple of nights in a row!

INGREDIENTS | SERVES 6–8

15 ounces dried black beans

15 ounces dried kidney beans

15 ounces dried garbanzo beans

15 ounces dried white beans

2 cups Tasty Tomato Sauce (see recipe in Chapter 4)

2 cups chopped Roma tomatoes

2 cups fresh or frozen corn kernels

1 yellow onion, chopped

1 celery stalk, chopped

1 green pepper, chopped

4 tablespoons Italian seasoning

1 tablespoon cayenne pepper

1. Soak all beans for 24 hours, rinse, and drain.

2. In a cold slow cooker, combine all ingredients.

3. Set slow cooker to low.

4. Cook for 8–10 hours, or until ingredients are soft and flavors well blended.

PER SERVING Calories: 662.24 | Fat: 4.97 g | Protein: 39.48 g | Sodium: 522.50 mg | Fiber: 38.56 g | Carbohydrates: 121.5 g | Sugar: 28.704 g

That Beautiful Bean That Looks Like a Kidney

Everybody knows that beans are great sources of protein and fiber, but not too many know what that means. These tasty little morsels are extremely inexpensive, can be soaked overnight, and cooked up in a wide variety of ways with a vast number of recipes as limitless as the imagination. The fiber contained in beans like the kidney variety helps to maintain optimal blood pressure, regulate blood sugar levels, and keep the food in your digestive tract moving right along.

Sautéed Spinach, Mushrooms, and Potatoes

Not many vegetables can compare to the iron-rich spinach leaves, which are as beautiful as they are tasty. Perfect for a busy weeknight!

INGREDIENTS | SERVES 4

5 red potatoes, cut into ¼" chunks

1 cup filtered water

1 tablespoon minced garlic

1 cup sliced portabella mushrooms

3 cups whole baby spinach leaves

2 teaspoons garlic powder

1 teaspoon freshly ground black pepper

1 teaspoon all-natural sea salt

1. In a large skillet over medium to medium-high heat, combine the potatoes, water, and minced garlic and bring to a simmer for about 7–10 minutes or until potatoes are fork-tender.

2. Move the potatoes from the skillet to a mixing bowl or large dish, and return skillet to heat with olive oil spray.

3. Add the mushrooms to the skillet and sauté until softened. Add the spinach leaves and fold until soft, about 2–3 minutes.

4. Combine the mushrooms and spinach with the potatoes, mix in seasonings, and blend well.

PER SERVING Calories: 202.78 | Fat: 0.467 g | Protein: 5.995 g | Sodium: 628.34 mg | Fiber: 7.48 g | Carbohydrates: 45.54 g | Sugar: 3.75 g

Great Fakeout Meatballs

Although meatballs are normally packed with meat, vegetarians should be able to enjoy this classic Italian dish, too. This alternative recipe combines loads of vegetables and healthy grains for dense, and scrumptious, meatballs that will become a family favorite.

INGREDIENTS | SERVES 4

1 zucchini, minced

½ eggplant, minced

1 yellow onion, minced

1 cup mushrooms, minced

2 slices sprouted grain bread

1 container firm tofu

3 teaspoons Italian seasoning

3 teaspoons garlic powder

2 teaspoons freshly ground black pepper

1 teaspoon all-natural sea salt

Substitutes for Processed Breadcrumbs

There's no doubt about it, having a food processor or high-speed blender just makes life easier. When you need fresh breadcrumbs, but don't want the store-bought versions that are loaded with sodium, fat, calories, and preservatives, all you have to do is throw some healthy whole grain, whole wheat bread slices in the processor or blender and reduce to crumbs. You can use them fresh, allow them to get stale (about 2–3 hours), or bake them on a foil-lined pan for 15–20 minutes. They're a delicious, healthy alternative to store-bought breadcrumbs.

1. Sauté the minced zucchini, eggplant, onion, and mushrooms until extremely soft.

2. In a food processor, reduce the bread slices to breadcrumbs.

3. Add the tofu, sautéed vegetables, and seasonings to the bread and process until well-blended.

4. Preheat oven to 350°F, and cover a baking sheet with foil and spray with olive oil.

5. Form the mixture into balls and line up evenly on the baking sheet.

6. Bake for 25–30 minutes, or until completely cooked through.

PER SERVING Calories: 113.49 | Fat: 2.81 g | Protein: 9.03 g | Sodium: 679.58 mg | Fiber: 3.75 g | Carbohydrates: 14.75 g | Sugar: 4.51 g

Wild Mushroom Risotto

This delicious blend of mushrooms, sautéed onions and garlic, and long-grain brown rice make for a splendid dish of tasty risotto. Slightly stickier than traditional brown rice, this is one pot of scrumptiousness.

INGREDIENTS | SERVES 2

1 tablespoon olive oil

1 yellow onion, minced

2 tablespoons minced garlic

1⅓ cups long-grain brown rice

3¾ cups filtered water

6 cups baby portabella mushrooms, quartered

1 teaspoon all-natural sea salt

1 teaspoon freshly ground black pepper

2 teaspoons Italian seasoning

Risotto's Bad Rap

Many people don't make their own risotto because it's rumored to be so difficult: too wet, too dry, too sticky, or not sticky enough. But just stir constantly, use fresh ingredients, and watch closely for all the water to be absorbed, and you'll create a delicious risotto every time.

1. Drizzle the olive oil in a saucepan over medium heat, and sauté the minced onion and garlic until softened, about 5 minutes.

2. Add the uncooked rice to the saucepan and turn to coat in the oil, garlic, and onions. Stir over heat for 2 minutes.

3. Add the water, mushrooms, and seasonings to the saucepan, and stir to combine.

4. Bring to a boil, reduce heat to low, and simmer uncovered for 20 minutes, stirring frequently.

5. Risotto is done when the rice has absorbed all of the liquid, and is sticky but cooked through.

PER SERVING Calories: 612.35 | Fat: 11.18 g | Protein: 16.21 g | Sodium: 1224.75 mg | Fiber: 9.06 g | Carbohydrates: 115.11 g | Sugar: 8.87 g

Sweet Tofu with Summer Squash

Agave nectar sweetens up this meal for a surprising and satisfying flavor explosion. Just wait until you feast your eyes on this meal. It's as fun to look at as it is to eat!

INGREDIENTS | SERVES 2

1 tablespoon olive oil

1 pound summer squash, peeled and cut into ½" squares

3 tablespoons agave nectar, divided

1 container of extra-firm tofu, cut into thin strips

½ teaspoon nutmeg

½ teaspoon ginger

½ teaspoon cinnamon

1 teaspoon all-natural sea salt

1. Prepare a large skillet with the olive oil over medium heat.

2. Add the squash to the pan with 1 tablespoon of the agave, and sauté until tender, about 10 minutes.

3. Remove the squash from the skillet and place the tofu into the skillet with 1 tablespoon of agave. Sauté until slightly browned.

4. Return the squash to the skillet and combine with the tofu. Add the spices and remaining tablespoon of agave, and toss until squash and tofu are coated.

5. Remove from heat, plate, and serve immediately.

PER SERVING Calories: 266.47 | Fat: 11.53 g | Protein: 11.79 g | Sodium: 1241.07 mg | Fiber: 0.71 g | Carbohydrates: 31.28 g | Sugar: 28.43 g

CHAPTER 10

Scrumptious Sides

Mediterranean Couscous

Plain couscous is mighty tasty, but this recipe jazzes it up with even more flavor. It's an easy side dish for summer potlucks!

INGREDIENTS | SERVES 4

4 cups prepared couscous
1 tablespoon balsamic vinegar
1 roasted red pepper
½ cup steamed asparagus spears

1. After preparing couscous according to the instructions, pour into a large serving dish, and mix with the balsamic vinegar.

2. Mince the roasted red pepper and asparagus spears, and toss with the couscous.

PER SERVING Calories: 663.29 | Fat: 1.18 g | Protein: 22.72 g | Sodium: 19.44 mg | Fiber: 9.51 g | Carbohydrates: 139.66 g | Sugar: 1.63 g

Scalloped Tomatoes

This is a delicious way to prepare tomatoes. Not only is the presentation beautiful, with the vibrant colors of the tomatoes and the basil, but the aroma and taste are intoxicating!

INGREDIENTS | SERVES 4

4 large tomatoes
¼ cup basil leaves, measured then chopped
1 tablespoon olive oil
1 teaspoon garlic powder
1 teaspoon all-natural sea salt
1 teaspoon freshly ground black pepper

Olive Oil for a Longer Life

The Mediterranean population (which eats mostly extra-virgin olive oil) has shown to suffer from far less degenerative diseases like cancers and heart disease than the U.S. population (which uses primarily animal fats and butter). That's why scientists think that the type of fats used might be more important than the amount. Give olive oil a shot!

1. Preheat oven to 400°F, and prepare a casserole dish 9" x 9" with olive oil spray.

2. Slice the tomatoes to ¼" thickness, and layer in the casserole dish.

3. Sprinkle the basil leaves over the tomatoes and drizzle the olive oil over top. Season with the garlic powder, salt, and pepper.

4. Bake at 400°F for 20 minutes, or until soft and slightly crisp.

PER SERVING Calories: 34.12 | Fat: 3.41 g | Protein: 0.26 g | Sodium: 590.27 mg | Fiber: 0.25 g | Carbohydrates: 0.93 g | Sugar: 0.03 g

Loaded Baked Potatoes

Potatoes are an excellent source of abundant vitamins and minerals, such as vitamins C and B$_6$ and manganese, copper, and potassium. Topped with delicious clean toppings, these potatoes are a side dish that only taste like a guilty pleasure.

INGREDIENTS | SERVES 2

1 tablespoon olive oil

2 large Idaho potatoes, washed

2 teaspoons garlic powder

1½ teaspoons all-natural sea salt

1 teaspoon freshly ground black pepper

2 tablespoons plain nonfat yogurt

½ cup chopped scallions

Pass the Spuds, Please

Whether you bake, roast, sauté, or mash these tasty root vegetables, they're not difficult to whip into a delicious dish. Loaded with tons of fiber and complex carbohydrates, and low in calories and fat, potatoes have gotten a bad reputation because of how they're traditionally served. Potatoes are an amazing source of well-rounded nutrition that makes for a great main course or accompaniment, but if loaded with heavy cream, lots of butter, excess salt, and bacon, there's not much room to call them anything but unhealthy. Stripped down or loaded up with fresh natural ingredients, spuds are a star that should be enjoyed and recognized for what they are . . . delicious nutrition!

1. Preheat oven to 400°F.

2. Drizzle the olive oil over the potatoes and coat with your hands.

3. Sprinkle the garlic powder and 1 teaspoon of salt all over the skins of the potatoes.

4. Place the potatoes on the oven's middle grate, and bake for 45–60 minutes, or until the outsides are crispy and they give when pressed on the sides.

5. Let cool for about 5 minutes, and slit on the top. Press the ends slightly to make the slit open.

6. Sprinkle the remaining ½ teaspoon of sea salt and black pepper in the two openings. Spoon the yogurt in the openings, and top with the chopped scallions.

PER SERVING Calories: 253.03 | Fat: 7.55 g | Protein: 5.79 g | Sodium: 23.11 mg | Fiber: 3.45 g | Carbohydrates: 42.62 g | Sugar: 3.29 g

Mashed Sweet Potatoes

Sweet potatoes have a beautiful flavor that you can brighten even more with the simple addition of cinnamon and nutmeg. This recipe uses vanilla almond milk to create a creamy texture, so there's no need for heavy butter or cream.

INGREDIENTS | SERVES 4

2 large sweet potatoes
1 cup vanilla almond milk
1 teaspoon cinnamon
1 teaspoon nutmeg

No Vitamin A Supplement Needed

Sweet potatoes are beautiful, naturally sweet versions of the much-loved potato. Packed with lycopene and carotenoids, these amazing spuds are also abundant in vitamin A. Amazingly, just one single sweet potato carries less than one hundred calories, but boasts more than two-and-a-half times the daily recommended amount of vitamin A. Just one sweet potato can reduce inflammation, protect against free radical damage, and supply an enormous amount of vitamin A!

1. Peel the potatoes, and slice into ½"-slices.

2. Rinse the sweet potatoes and place in a pot. Cover the potatoes with water and set the pot over medium-high heat for 20–30 minutes, or until potatoes are fork-tender.

3. Remove from the heat, drain, and move the potatoes to a serving dish.

4. Mash the potatoes, and gradually add the almond milk until the desired consistency is achieved.

5. Season with the cinnamon and nutmeg to taste, stir, and serve.

PER SERVING Calories: 70.26 | Fat: 0.25 g | Protein: 1.33 g | Sodium: 80.9 mg | Fiber: 2.62 g | Carbohydrates: 13.82 g | Sugar: 2.90 g

Spicy Broccolini

Not too many people think of broccolini as a go-to veggie, but this is one healthy little morsel that deserves attention. This simple side dish can accent all types of meals like chicken, fish, meat, or vegetarian dishes.

INGREDIENTS | SERVES 2

1 tablespoon olive oil
1 tablespoon chopped garlic
1 pound broccolini
1 teaspoon all-natural sea salt
1 teaspoon red pepper flakes

What Is Broccolini?

A part of the broccoli family (just a baby version of it), broccolini is a delicious vegetable that many eat raw. Find the gorgeous, long-stemmed variety in your grocer's fresh vegetable section and at many produce stands.

1. In a large skillet over medium heat, drizzle the tablespoon of olive oil and sauté the garlic for about a minute.

2. Add the broccolini, sea salt, and red pepper flakes to the garlic and continue to sauté for 3–5 minutes.

3. Once the broccolini is slightly softened, but still crisp, remove from heat and plate.

PER SERVING Calories: 144.97 | Fat: 7.75 g | Protein: 6.69 g | Sodium: 1253.93 mg | Fiber: 6.15 g | Carbohydrates: 16.78 g | Sugar: 3.94 g

Perfect Acorn Squash Cups

This is a delicious recipe that also makes for a beautiful presentation at a dinner party. These tender and delicious acorn squash cups provide perfectly portioned individual servings.

INGREDIENTS | SERVES 1

1 large acorn squash
1 tablespoon olive oil
1 tablespoon agave nectar
1 teaspoon cinnamon
1 teaspoon all-natural sea salt

1. Preheat an oven to 375°F. Cut the squash in half, and remove seeds and pulp.

2. Place the squash in a roasting pan with the hollowed insides facing up. Coat the cut top edges and insides of the squash halves with the olive oil, drizzle the insides with the agave nectar, and sprinkle the cinnamon and salt on the top edges and insides of both.

3. Bake at 375 for 30–45 minutes, or until the insides of the squash are fork-tender.

PER SERVING Calories: 361.75 | Fat: 13.96 g | Protein: 3.60 g | Sodium: 2372.05 mg | Fiber: 7.71 g | Carbohydrates: 64.20 g | Sugar: 17.45 g

Stuffed Mushrooms

These delicious mushrooms can be the perfect appetizer or side dish. Pairing perfectly with fish, meat, vegetables, or pasta, this is a versatile recipe that is quick, easy, and heavenly.

INGREDIENTS | SERVES 6

12 large white mushrooms
½ small zucchini
½ red pepper
1 teaspoon garlic powder
1 tablespoon filtered water
¼ cup crumbled goat cheese

What Makes Goat Cheese Superior?

If you're wondering why goat cheese is "clean" but pasteurized processed cheese isn't, it is because of the drastically different makeup of the cheeses. Goat's milk is far superior to that of a cow because there is no need to homogenize goat milk. Goat's milk is naturally homogenized, while cow's milk must be homogenized in the manufacturing process. Without mechanical homogenization, valuable nutrition remains intact and the resulting product has shown to be far less irritating to the human digestive system and allergenic. In fact, even some lactose-intolerant people are able to consume it without problems.

1. Clean the mushrooms with a dry paper towel; remove and reserve stems.

2. Mince the zucchini, red pepper, and mushroom stems.

3. Prepare a skillet with olive oil spray over medium heat, and add the zucchini and red pepper. Sautee for about 2–3 minutes, and add mushroom stems and garlic powder and continue to sauté until all veggies are tender.

4. Add water to skillet as needed to prevent sticking and promote steaming.

5. Remove sautéed veggies from heat and stuff mushroom caps full with the mixture.

6. Preheat oven to 375°F and use a small grate to place the mushrooms on in the oven.

7. Place the crumbled goat cheese in the tops, and bake for 20 minutes.

PER SERVING Calories: 56.41 | Fat: 3.52 g | Protein: 4.32 g | Sodium: 36.05 mg | Fiber: 0.73 g | Carbohydrates: 2.68 g | Sugar: 1.57 g

Zucchini Boats

Zucchini is a versatile vegetable that takes on whatever flavors it's combined with. This beautiful presentation of zucchini uses all-natural ingredients to create a delicious dish with vibrant colors and flavors for a tasty snack or side.

INGREDIENTS | SERVES 4

4 large zucchini

1 red pepper, minced

1 red onion, minced

1 cup mushrooms, minced

1 teaspoon garlic powder

1 teaspoon all-natural sea salt

1 teaspoon freshly ground black pepper

1 cup crumbled goat cheese

1. Preheat oven to 400°F and prepare a small oven grate with olive oil spray.

2. Cut the zucchini in half lengthwise, and clean the seeds out of the center to make a large opening for the vegetables.

3. Prepare a large skillet with olive oil spray over medium heat.

4. Sauté the pepper, onion, and mushrooms with the garlic powder, salt, and pepper until veggies are slightly softened.

5. Pack the sautéed veggies into the centers of each zucchini, and top with the goat cheese.

6. Bake directly on the oven grate at 400°F for 20 minutes, or until zucchini is tender and cheese is melted.

PER SERVING Calories: 310.92 | Fat: 20.72 g | Protein: 20.74 g | Sodium: 802.41 mg | Fiber: 3.31 g | Carbohydrates: 12.69 g | Sugar: 8.36 g

Peppers and Pasta

Whip up this recipe instead of a boxed pasta salad the next time you have to bring a side dish to a cookout. The colored peppers make for a feast for your eyes and your mouth!

INGREDIENTS | SERVES 2

1 red pepper, top and ribs removed and cut into thin strips

1 green pepper, top and ribs removed and cut into thin strips

1 yellow pepper, top and ribs removed and cut into thin strips

1 tablespoon filtered water

2 cups 100% whole wheat fettuccine, cooked

1 tablespoon olive oil

1 teaspoon garlic powder

1 teaspoon onion powder

1 teaspoon all-natural sea salt

1 teaspoon freshly ground black pepper

1. Prepare a large skillet with olive oil spray over medium heat, and add peppers to the hot skillet.

2. Sauté the peppers until tender and still crisp, adding water as needed to prevent sticking.

3. Pour the cooked pasta into a large bowl, and add sautéed peppers. Add the tablespoon of olive oil, garlic powder, onion powder, salt, and pepper, and toss to coat.

4. Serve immediately.

PER SERVING Calories: 327.85 | Fat: 8.41 g | Protein: 10.12 g | Sodium: 1188.15 mg | Fiber: 6.14 g | Carbohydrates: 54.11 g | Sugar: 5.19 g

"Lighten Up" Potato Salad

Most people love potato salad, but avoid it because of the fat and calories.
This recipe makes the classic delicious dish healthy and nutritious.

INGREDIENTS | SERVES 4

6 red potatoes, cut into ½" cubes
¾ cup celery, chopped
¾ cup chopped scallions
1 cup plain nonfat yogurt
1 teaspoon garlic powder
1 teaspoon all-natural sea salt
1 teaspoon freshly ground black pepper
3 hard-boiled eggs

Substitutions You'd Barely Notice

If you're in charge of the potato salad at your next get-together, try some healthy substitutions that your friends may not even notice. Traditional potato salad is packed with fat, calories, sugar, and sodium from preservative-packed ingredients like mayonnaise, bacon, and relish. Instead, use only fresh ingredients that specifically contribute to the taste, texture, flavor, and nutritional value.

1. Place potatoes in a pot, cover with water, and bring to a boil over medium-high heat for 10 minutes, or until the potatoes are fork-tender.

2. Remove the potatoes, drain, and set aside to cool.

3. In a large bowl, combine the celery, scallions, yogurt, and seasonings, and mix well.

4. Peel the eggs, discard the shells and yolks, and chop the egg whites.

5. Add the chopped egg whites and potatoes to the yogurt mixture and toss to coat.

6. Refrigerate for 1 hour, and enjoy!

PER SERVING Calories: 323.58 | Fat: 6.18 g | Protein: 12.71 g | Sodium: 710.64 mg | Fiber: 8.56 g | Carbohydrates: 55.90 g | Sugar: 8.14 g

Garlic Mashed Potatoes

Using almond milk and delicious spices, this heart-healthy, waistline-friendly recipe lightens up the traditional dish with the same amazing flavors.

INGREDIENTS | SERVES 4

2 large Idaho potatoes, cut into ½" slices (leave skin on if you prefer)

2 tablespoons minced garlic

1 cup unsweetened almond milk

1 teaspoon all-natural sea salt

1 teaspoon freshly ground black pepper

Ahhh, Garlic!

Traditional dishes that are normally prepared with butter, salt, and additional fattening ingredients can be made healthier and more appealing by eliminating poor ingredients and adding healthy ingredients that add tons of flavor naturally . . . like garlic.

1. Place potatoes in a pot of water with the minced garlic.

2. Bring the potatoes to a boil over medium heat, and cook for 10–15 minutes, or until the potatoes are soft.

3. Remove the potatoes and garlic from the heat, drain, and pour into a large mixing bowl.

4. Add the almond milk gradually while mashing, and season with salt and pepper to taste.

PER SERVING Calories: 101.83 | Fat: 0.12 g | Protein: 2.86 g | Sodium: 640.73 mg | Fiber: 1.87 g | Carbohydrates: 21.0 g | Sugar: 0.71 g

Broccoli-Cauliflower Bake

Fibrous veggies are an important part of any diet, but most people don't eat enough. This recipe is packed with two favorites—broccoli and cauliflower—and combines them with delicious goat cheese for a flavorful dish brimming with excellent taste and nutrition.

INGREDIENTS | SERVES 4

1 pound broccoli florets

1 pound cauliflower florets

2 tablespoons olive oil

1 cup crumbled goat cheese

1. Preheat an oven to 375°F and prepare a 9" x 13" casserole dish with olive oil spray.

2. In a large mixing bowl, combine the broccoli and cauliflower with the olive oil and goat cheese. Mix to coat.

3. Pour the mixture into the casserole dish, and bake for 30–45 minutes, or until the vegetables are tender and the cheese is melted.

PER SERVING Calories: 378.87 | Fat: 27.41 g | Protein: 22.4 g | Sodium: 264.46 mg | Fiber: 5.15 g | Carbohydrates: 14.22 g | Sugar: 5.26 g

Scalloped Potatoes with Leeks and Olives

Scalloped potatoes are traditionally packed with cheese and heavy cream. Just as tasty, but with a fraction of the fat, calories, sodium, and dairy, these scalloped potatoes join forces with crunchy leeks and naturally salty olives for a taste sensation that is out of this world!

INGREDIENTS | SERVES 6

4 Idaho potatoes, sliced into ⅛" rounds

2 leeks, cut into ¼" pieces

1 cup sliced green olives

1 tablespoon olive oil

1 teaspoon garlic powder

1 teaspoon freshly ground black pepper

1. Prepare a 9" x 13" baking dish with olive oil spray, and preheat the oven to 375°F.

2. In a large mixing bowl, combine the potato slices, leeks, and sliced olives with the olive oil, and pour into the baking dish.

3. Season with the garlic and pepper, and bake for 30–45 minutes.

PER SERVING Calories: 144.29 | Fat: 2.64 g | Protein: 3.14 g | Sodium: 210.22 mg | Fiber: 4.80 g | Carbohydrates: 28.48 g | Sugar: 2.80 g

Carrot Coleslaw

The sweetness of the agave and raisins and the crunch of the carrots make for an unique combination of textures and flavors in a light and creamy sauce. Perfect for a summer picnic!

INGREDIENTS | SERVES 4

1 pound carrots, cut into matchsticks

1 cup no-sugar-added raisins

½ cup plain nonfat yogurt

1 tablespoon agave nectar

1 teaspoon all-natural sea salt

1. In a large mixing bowl, combine the carrots, raisins, and yogurt with the agave nectar, and mix to coat.

2. Season with the teaspoon of salt, and blend well.

PER SERVING Calories: 190.18 | Fat: 1.43 g | Protein: 3.35 g | Sodium: 685.37 mg | Fiber: 4.60 g | Carbohydrates: 45.35 g | Sugar: 32.54 g

Perfect Polenta

This is a great dish for promoting energy without weighing you down. Thick and hearty, yet light and delicious, this recipe can be transformed into just about anything. You can make it into cakes, roll it up and slice it, or just enjoy it with a spoon!

INGREDIENTS | SERVES 12

8½ cups filtered water

2 tablespoons extra-virgin olive oil

1 tablespoon all-natural sea salt

2 cups cornmeal

Polenta: It's What's for Dinner, or Lunch, or Breakfast, or a Snack!

Polenta is a low-fat, low-calorie dish that is delicious and versatile, but very few people enjoy it. When asked why they don't indulge in this tasty food that can be served in a million ways and at any meal-time, most people say they don't know how to make it. Yet it's absurdly easy to make! You can roll into a log and freeze for easy cuttings of the perfect portions, or you can just store it in an airtight container in your refrigerator for sampling any time of day.

1. Bring the water and olive oil to a boil in a large pot over medium heat, and season with the sea salt. Pour the cornmeal into the pot, and whisk vigorously to prevent clumping.

2. The polenta will become thick. Keep stirring for 25–30 minutes, or until it becomes extremely thick.

3. Remove the polenta from the heat, and move to a cold, covered glass bowl.

4. Let stand for 10–15 minutes, covered, and serve, or wrap and refrigerate for later use.

PER SERVING Calories: 104.76 | Fat: 2.66 g | Protein: 1.67 g | Sodium: 596.13 mg | Fiber: 0.92 g | Carbohydrates: 18.21 g | Sugar: 0.38 g

"Not Fried" Fried Rice

This side dish is a cleaned-up version of the popular Chinese takeout menu option. Delicious and nutritious brown rice is cooked with sautéed onions, scrambled eggs, sweet peas, and salty soy sauce for restaurant-taste with homemade nutrition.

INGREDIENTS | SERVES 4

½ yellow onion, minced

2 eggs, beaten

1 cup baby sweet peas

2 cups cooked brown rice

1 cup carrot, cut into matchsticks

1 tablespoon low-sodium soy sauce

Way Better than Takeout

Homemade "fried" rice is not only simple, but it's packed with natural vegetables and tons of flavor from spices. If you decide to get real fried rice from a restaurant, you can bet the rice is white and nutrition-depleted, the vegetables are not fresh, and the seasonings used are most likely not sodium- and sugar-conscious.

1. Prepare a large skillet with olive oil spray over medium heat, and sauté the minced onion.

2. Pour in the beaten eggs, and scramble until lightly fluffy. Break up the eggs into small pieces.

3. Add the peas and carrots to heat through, and remove the skillet from the heat.

4. Pour the rice in a large mixing bowl, and add the onions, eggs, carrots, and peas. Blend well.

5. Drizzle the soy sauce over the rice, and toss to coat completely.

PER SERVING Calories: 163.84 | Fat: 3.38 g | Protein: 6.06 g | Sodium: 280.10 mg | Fiber: 2.79 g | Carbohydrates: 27.34 g | Sugar: 2.15 g

Perfect Potato Fries

Served with the perfect hamburger (or portabella burger), these fries make for a healthy spin on the traditional storebought or restaurant-ordered variety. Baking versus frying is always a smart trade-up, so these fries are the perfect accompaniment to any meal.

INGREDIENTS | SERVES 4

6 Idaho potatoes, washed
1 tablespoon olive oil
1 teaspoon all-natural sea salt
1 teaspoon freshly ground black pepper
1 teaspoon paprika

1. Preheat oven to 400°F and line a baking sheet with aluminum foil.

2. Cut the potatoes in half lengthwise, then in long strips about ¼"–½" in width.

3. In a large resealable plastic bag, toss the potatoes with the olive oil to coat.

4. In a small dish, combine the salt, pepper, and paprika.

5. Place the potato strips on the baking sheet and sprinkle with half of the seasonings. Bake for 15–20 minutes, or until crispy.

6. Turn the fries to bake the opposite sides, and sprinkle with remaining seasonings. Return to the oven and continue baking about 15 minutes, or until golden brown and crispy.

PER SERVING Calories: 285.26 | Fat: 3.72 g | Protein: 6.98 g | Sodium: 605.92 mg | Fiber: 4.51 g | Carbohydrates: 58.4 g | Sugar: 2.04 g

Ultimate Spinach and Mushroom Risotto

This delicious risotto is beautiful and amazingly tasty. Sticky long-grain rice makes for a delightfully light yet hearty background to the fresh vegetable additions.

INGREDIENTS | SERVES 2

1 tablespoon olive oil

1 yellow onion, minced

2 tablespoons minced garlic

1⅓ cups long-grain brown rice

3¾ cups filtered water

6 cups baby portabella mushrooms, quartered

1 teaspoon all-natural sea salt

1 teaspoon freshly ground black pepper

2 teaspoons Italian seasoning

2 cups baby spinach, chopped

1. Drizzle the olive oil in a saucepan over medium heat, and sauté the minced onion and garlic until softened, about 5 minutes.

2. Add the uncooked rice to the saucepan and turn to coat in the oil, garlic, and onions. Stir over heat for 2 minutes.

3. Add the water, mushrooms, and seasonings to the saucepan, and stir to combine.

4. Bring to a boil, reduce heat to low, and simmer uncovered for 20 minutes, stirring frequently.

5. Risotto is done when the rice has absorbed all of the liquid, and is sticky but cooked through. Fold in the chopped spinach, and stir over heat until the spinach is wilted and combined throughout, about 1–2 minutes.

PER SERVING Calories: 619.25 | Fat: 11.30 g | Protein: 17.06 g | Sodium: 1235.13 mg | Fiber: 9.72 g | Carbohydrates: 116.19 g | Sugar: 9 g

Quinoa with Mixed Vegetables

*As a unique side dish, or a new and exciting entrée, this quinoa recipe
is a quick and easy solution to any dinnertime dilemma.*

INGREDIENTS | SERVES 2

1 cup dry organic quinoa

2 cups filtered water

½ tablespoon garlic powder

½ tablespoon onion powder

½ red onion, chopped

1 cup broccoli florets

1 tablespoon extra-virgin olive oil

1 cup portabella mushrooms

1 teaspoon all-natural sea salt

1. Rinse the quinoa thoroughly, and combine with the water in a medium saucepan over medium heat and bring to a boil. Reduce heat to low, add half of the garlic powder and onion powder, and simmer for 15 minutes.

2. In a large sauté pan over medium heat, sauté the onion and broccoli in the olive oil for 7–10 minutes or until all are slightly softened.

3. Add the mushrooms and remaining half of the garlic and onion powders to the sauté pan and continue cooking until all veggies are soft.

4. Remove the quinoa from the heat and transfer to a separate dish. Add the sautéed vegetables, and sprinkle with salt to taste.

PER SERVING Calories: 408.4 | Fat: 12.256 g | Protein: 14.495 g | Sodium: 1203.259 mg | Fiber: 8.159 g | Carbohydrates: 61.79 g | Sugar: 3.014 g

Cold Quinoa Salad

Mixed with cool cucumbers and chilled chicken, then blended with olive oil and vinegar, this quinoa-based salad blends textures and flavors for a delightful meal or snack option any time of day.

INGREDIENTS | SERVES 2

1 cup dry organic quinoa

2 cups filtered water

1 English cucumber, chopped

1 grilled boneless, skinless chicken breast, cooled and chopped

1½ tablespoons red wine vinegar

1½ tablespoons balsamic vinegar

1 teaspoon garlic powder

1 teaspoon onion powder

Quinoa for Headache Relief

Many headache sufferers would benefit greatly from an increase in magnesium in their diet. Shown to reduce the frequency and intensity of headaches by allowing the blood vessels of the body to relax, magnesium may be the ticket to headache-free days. So eat your quinoa—since it contains almost half of the recommended daily value of magnesium in just ¼ cup!

1. Rinse the quinoa thoroughly, and combine with the water in a medium saucepan over medium heat, and bring to a boil. Reduce heat to low, add the garlic powder and onion powder, and simmer for 15 minutes.

2. Remove the quinoa from the heat, transfer to a separate dish, and fluff with a fork. Allow to cool.

3. Add the chopped cucumber and chicken to the quinoa and toss to combine.

4. Drizzle the salad with the vinegars and toss to coat completely.

5. Cover and refrigerate the salad for 1 hour, or more, to allow the flavors to marry.

PER SERVING Calories: 415.175 | Fat: 7.138 g | Protein: 27.841 g | Sodium: 88.46 mg | Fiber: 6.703 g | Carbohydrates: 59.999 g | Sugar: 2.513 g

Roasted Red Potatoes and Onions

Roasted vegetables go great as a side to almost any main dish. These beautiful red potatoes are intensified with the crisp crunch of red onions, and then heightened in flavor with the aromatic addition of garlic and turmeric.

INGREDIENTS | SERVES 4

8 red potatoes, cubed into 1" pieces

2 red onions, cut into 1" chunks

1 tablespoon olive oil

2 teaspoons garlic powder

1 teaspoon all-natural sea salt

1 teaspoon freshly ground black pepper

½ teaspoon turmeric

Texture for Satiety

Many people reach for something with a crunch when they're hungry. The average person probably reaches for potato chips or crunchy cookies rather than a healthy treat. Crazy sounding, but true: The crunch of celery, carrots, or other fruits and veggies with a crisp texture may be all you need . . . so put the cookies and chips away.

1. Preheat oven to 400°F, and spray a 9" x 13" baking dish with olive oil spray.

2. In a large resealable plastic bag, combine the potatoes and onions with the olive oil.

3. Sprinkle in the garlic powder, salt, pepper, and turmeric, and toss to coat.

4. Pour the potatoes and onion with the olive oil from the bag into the baking dish, and bake for 45 minutes, or until potatoes are crispy on the outside and fork-tender inside.

PER SERVING Calories: 352.77 | Fat: 3.91 g | Protein: 8.07 g | Sodium: 618.45 mg | Fiber: 11.49 g | Carbohydrates: 73.61 g | Sugar: 7.28 g

CHAPTER 11

Satisfying Soups

Amazing Minestrone

Minestrone is, in theory, a healthy soup. But many canned versions are loaded with salt and veggies that aren't fresh. By using all fresh and natural ingredients, though, you can optimize the quality of the vitamin and mineral content in the veggies and, thus, the soup.

INGREDIENTS | SERVES 8

4 tablespoons olive oil

5 garlic cloves

2 yellow onions, chopped

2 cups chopped celery

2 cups chopped carrots

4 cups filtered water

4 cups Tasty Tomato Sauce (see recipe in Chapter 4)

2 zucchini, chopped

2 cups green beans, chopped

1 cup soaked kidney beans

1 cup soaked white beans

2 cups baby spinach leaves

1 tablespoon oregano

2 tablespoons chopped basil

1 teaspoon all-natural sea salt

1 teaspoon freshly ground black pepper

1. In a large pot over medium heat, sauté 1 tablespoon of olive oil, garlic, onion, celery, and carrots for 8–10 minutes.

2. Add the water and the tomato sauce to the pot, and bring to a boil.

3. Reduce heat to low and add the zucchini, green beans, kidney beans, white beans, spinach leaves, and spices. Simmer on low for 1–2 hours.

4. Serve the soup by itself or over cooked whole wheat shell pasta.

PER SERVING Calories: 282.81 | Fat: 7.59 g | Protein: 13.50 g | Sodium: 1002.04 mg | Fiber: 14.70 g | Carbohydrates: 43.85 g | Sugar: 11.60 g

Satisfying Soup for Pick-Me-Up Snacks

Indulging in a hot bowl of soup rich in vegetables, specialty spices, and fresh ingredients can actually make for a satisfying meal that will keep you feeling fresh and rejuvenated while also curbing cravings and keeping a sensation of satiety. Whether it's a morning snack, a light lunch, or a hearty supper, don't be afraid to make soup the star meal (or snack!) of the day.

Classic Tomato Soup

*With canned tomato soup containing absurd amounts of sodium—and even sugar—
this is a refreshing homemade version that's super tasty and healthy.*

INGREDIENTS | SERVES 4

1 cup filtered water

10 tomatoes

1 cup chopped basil

1 tablespoon minced garlic

2 teaspoons all-natural sea salt

2 cups Tasty Tomato Sauce (see recipe in Chapter 4)

1 cup plain Greek-style yogurt

1. In a large pot, bring the water, tomatoes, basil, and garlic to a boil. Reduce heat to low and simmer for about 15–20 minutes. Allow to cool.

2. With an immersion blender, emulsify the tomatoes and spices completely until no bits remain.

3. Add the sea salt, all of the Tasty Tomato Sauce, and the yogurt ¼ cup at a time, and use the immersion blender to fully combine. Serve hot or cold.

PER SERVING Calories: 127.0 | Fat: 0.91 g | Protein: 11.36 g | Sodium: 1867.98 mg | Fiber: 5.74 g | Carbohydrates: 22.17 g | Sugar: 15.81 g

White Bean Wonder

Beautiful and tasty, this simple recipe is a great dish for a snack or supper, served hot or cold.

INGREDIENTS | SERVES 4

2 cups filtered water

2 cups Tasty Tomato Sauce (see recipe in Chapter 4)

1 cup crushed tomatoes

2 garlic cloves, minced

1 cup soaked white beans

1 cup baby spinach

½ cup basil, chopped

1. In a large pot over medium heat, bring the water, tomato sauce, crushed tomatoes, and garlic to a boil.

2. Add the white beans, and reduce heat to low. Simmer for 10–15 minutes.

3. Add the spinach leaves and basil to the soup, and stir.

PER SERVING Calories: 193.09 | Fat: 0.69 g | Protein: 12.04 g | Sodium: 662.10 mg | Fiber: 11.11 g | Carbohydrates: 37.47 g | Sugar: 10.24 g

Fresh Forms of Fiber

You're adding powerful fiber to your diet with this soup. Combining soaked dried beans and fresh vegetables in a soup makes for a double dose of fiber.

Creamy Asparagus

Creamy soups are usually laden with fat and calories. Clean eating to the rescue! This version is just as tasty and has the same consistency . . . but has much less fat and fewer calories!

INGREDIENTS | SERVES 4

1 tablespoon olive oil
1 garlic clove
2 small Idaho potatoes, peeled and chopped
2 tablespoons filtered water
2 pounds asparagus, chopped
3 leeks, cleaned and chopped
2 teaspoons freshly ground black pepper
2 cups almond milk

1. In a stockpot over medium heat, sauté the olive oil, garlic, and potatoes for about 10–15 minutes, adding water as needed to prevent sticking and promote steaming.

2. Add asparagus, leeks, and pepper to the potatoes, and sauté until tender.

3. Add the almond milk to the pot and bring to a boil. Reduce heat to low and simmer for 10–15 minutes.

4. With an immersion blender, emulsify the ingredients until thick and creamy.

PER SERVING Calories: 212.67 | Fat: 3.99 g | Protein: 8.38 g | Sodium: 115.11 mg | Fiber: 9.26 g | Carbohydrates: 35.81 g | Sugar: 8.05 g

Green Chickpea Soup

Getting its green color from the spinach, broccoli, and leeks,
this soup gives green pea soup a run for its money!

INGREDIENTS | SERVES 4

4 cups filtered water

1 cup broccoli spears, chopped

1 leek, cleaned and chopped

2 cups soaked chickpeas

4 garlic cloves, finely minced

2 cups spinach leaves, chopped

1 teaspoon freshly ground black pepper

No Need for Store-Bought Stocks

If you're searching the grocer's aisles for boxed or canned stocks that deliver great taste with nutritional value and a short list of ingredients, good luck! Don't fret, though, because homemade stocks that are perfect starts to delicious soups are fast, easy, and inexpensive. By starting out with a pot full of a few more cups of water than you'll need for your soup, a ton of mixed vegetables and spices like onions, garlic, rosemary, basil, chives, tarragon, peppers, etc., you can infuse the water with the flavors by simmering the combination for an hour. Once the stock tastes like the perfect starter for your soup, strain the flavoring vegetables out, or keep them in for additional ingredients for your tasty soup blend.

1. In a large pot over medium heat, bring the water, broccoli, leek, chickpeas, and garlic to a boil. Reduce heat to low and simmer 15–20 minutes.

2. Add the spinach leaves and black pepper, and continue to cook for about 5 minutes. Remove from heat.

3. With an immersion blender, emulsify the ingredients until well-blended, and no bits remain.

PER SERVING Calories: 394.59 | Fat: 6.28 g | Protein: 20.95 g | Sodium: 55.66 mg | Fiber: 18.93 g | Carbohydrates: 67.19 g | Sugar: 12.05 g

Creamy Mushroom and Rice

Comfort food in a bowl is delivered piping hot with this recipe. Packed with delicious and nutritious mushrooms and brown rice, this soup gets its smooth creaminess from the protein-packed Greek-style yogurt. Brimming with healthy ingredients, and yet so simple to make!

INGREDIENTS | SERVES 4

4 cups mushrooms, chopped

3 cups filtered water, divided

2 teaspoons minced garlic

2 teaspoons all-natural sea salt

3 teaspoons freshly ground black pepper

2 cups cooked brown rice

1 cup plain Greek-style yogurt

Hot or Cold, Soup Is Soup

There are two ways to enjoy soup: hot or cold. Depending upon the soup, you may have the luck of being able to enjoy it either way. No more is a delicious cup of creamy mushroom and rice limited to winter days. The hearty soups that were traditionally served as hot dishes can now be served chilled, and the opposite is true as well. If heated gazpacho is what you crave, heat it up. Eating soup should be a delicious experience tailored to your own tastes and preferences, so feel free to make it hot or make it cold.

1. In a large pot, sauté the mushrooms in 2–4 tablespoons of the water, and the garlic, salt, and pepper for about 5–8 minutes, or until tender.

2. Reduce heat to low, add remaining water, and simmer for about 8–10 minutes.

3. Remove from the heat, add the rice to the pot, and allow to cool.

4. Stir to combine, add the yogurt, and blend well.

PER SERVING Calories: 94.87 | Fat: 0.30 g | Protein: 15.55 g | Sodium: 1247.18 mg | Fiber: 1.15 g | Carbohydrates: 8.87 g | Sugar: 6.33 g

Scrumptious Sage and Squash

Combining the sweet scrumptiousness of squash with aromatic and tasty sage, this soup is a surefire hit. Completely void of poor ingredients that most canned varieties would include, this is a homemade delight that can be enjoyed any time of day . . . or night.

INGREDIENTS | SERVES 4

4 cups filtered water

3 cups cubed summer squash, peeled and seeds removed

2 teaspoons all-natural sea salt

½ cup dried sage leaves

Brighten Flavors with Spices

There are certain ingredients that are well-known for being brighteners of tastes and flavors. Spices like sage fall into this category. Summer squash is a delicious vegetable that has a light, buttery, nutty taste that improves dramatically when seasoned just right. Rather than opting for fresh, many herbs are actually more powerful in their dried versions, so in soups, opt for dried spices . . . unless it's a garnish.

1. Bring the water to a boil in a large pot over medium heat.

2. Reduce heat to low, add the squash, salt, and sage, and simmer for about 20–25 minutes, or until fork-tender.

3. Using an immersion blender, emulsify the squash and sage until no bits remain.

4. Serve hot or cold, and garnish with a dollop of nonfat yogurt or crumbled sage leaves.

PER SERVING Calories: 26.16 | Fat: 0.66 g | Protein: 1.45 g | Sodium: 1188.13 mg | Fiber: 2.54 g | Carbohydrates: 5.27 g | Sugar: 1.93 g

Gazpacho

This delicious soup is packed with fresh vegetables that carry a bite. Usually served cold, there's no resisting the natural goodness of this great veggie-packed soup.

INGREDIENTS | SERVES 4

2 cups Tasty Tomato Sauce (see recipe in Chapter 4)

2 cups filtered water

2 tomatoes, chopped

1 yellow onion, chopped

1 green pepper, chopped

½ cup scallions, chopped

1 English cucumber, chopped

2 cloves garlic, finely minced

2 tablespoons freshly squeezed lemon juice

2 tablespoons red wine vinegar

1 teaspoon dried basil

1 teaspoon dried thyme

1 teaspoon all-natural sea salt

1 teaspoon freshly ground black pepper

1. In a food processor, combine all ingredients and pulse until thoroughly blended and still slightly chunky.

2. Chill at least 2–4 hours, but overnight is best!

PER SERVING Calories: 79.30 | Fat: 0.63 g | Protein: 3.54 g | Sodium: 1246.10 mg | Fiber: 4.44 g | Carbohydrates: 17.89 g | Sugar: 10.76 g

Thick and Hearty Potato Broccoli

If you're looking for an amazing-tasting bowl of soup that's hearty enough to be a meal, you've found it with this recipe. You won't need anything besides these nutritious potatoes, delicious fibrous broccoli, creamy protein-packed almond milk, and Greek-style yogurt.

INGREDIENTS | SERVES 4

3 cups unsweetened almond milk

2 Idaho potatoes, peeled

1 pound broccoli florets

1 cup plain low-fat Greek-style yogurt

2 teaspoons all-natural sea salt

Broaden Your Definition of "Hearty"

Hearty bowls of soup don't have to be thick stews made of meat and thickly cut vegetables. By puréeing a blend of yogurt or milk with a combination of your favorite vegetables and ingredients, you can end up with a filling meal. Thick and hearty, or thinned and hearty, it's the vegetables and ingredients that make up your delicious soup that make it a "hearty" helping.

1. In a large pot over medium heat, bring the almond milk and potatoes to a boil. Reduce heat to low and simmer about 8–10 minutes.

2. Add broccoli, and continue to simmer for 8–10 minutes.

3. Remove from heat, and chill for 5 minutes.

4. Using an immersion blender, emulsify ingredients.

5. Add yogurt ¼ cup at a time, and continue blending with the immersion blender.

6. Add salt, blend well, and serve.

PER SERVING Calories: 178.21 | Fat: 0.52 g | Protein: 12.26 g | Sodium: 1386.50 mg | Fiber: 6.22 g | Carbohydrates: 26.71 g | Sugar: 5.60 g

Cream of Broccoli

Usually filled with fat and calories, this recipe gets a clean makeover with the help of some thick yogurt and almond milk.

INGREDIENTS | SERVES 4

3 cups unsweetened almond milk
2 teaspoons all-natural sea salt
2 teaspoons garlic powder
1 teaspoon freshly ground black pepper
2 pounds broccoli florets
1 cup plain low-fat Greek-style yogurt

1. In a large pot over medium heat, bring the almond milk, salt, garlic powder, pepper, and broccoli to a boil. Reduce heat to low and simmer about 10–12 minutes.

2. Remove from heat, and chill for 5 minutes. Using an immersion blender, emulsify the broccoli mixture until no bits remain.

3. Add yogurt ¼ cup at a time, and continue blending with the immersion blender until well blended. Serve hot or cold.

PER SERVING Calories: 148.80 | Fat: 0.86 g | Protein: 13.92 g | Sodium: 1418.14 mg | Fiber: 6.84 g | Carbohydrates: 18.78 g | Sugar: 6.31 g

Creamy Butternut Squash with Leeks

"Creamy" doesn't have to mean "filled with fat and empty calories," and you don't have to use heavy cream to make dishes delicious.

INGREDIENTS | SERVES 4

3 cups filtered water
3 cups cubed butternut squash, peeled and seeds removed
2 cups cleaned leeks, chopped
2 teaspoons dried rosemary
1½ cups plain nonfat yogurt

1. In a large pot over medium heat, combine the water, squash, and leeks and bring to a boil. Reduce heat and simmer for 25–30 minutes.

2. Remove from heat and add rosemary. Use an immersion blender to emulsify the squash and leeks until smooth, with no bits remaining.

3. Add the nonfat yogurt ¼ cup at a time while blending until desired color, thickness, and creaminess is achieved.

PER SERVING Calories: 132.26 | Fat: 3.31 g | Protein: 4.93 g | Sodium: 60.97 mg | Fiber: 3.14 g | Carbohydrates: 23.21 g | Sugar: 8.33 g

Split Pea

Split pea soup is a classic favorite, but can be a completely unhealthy fat trap. Traditionally gaining a majority of its flavor from a ham bone, this recipe has been revamped and given a clean makeover with natural ingredients and home-soaked split peas, hold the hambone!

INGREDIENTS | SERVES 6

5 cups filtered water

2 cups dried split peas

1 cup celery, chopped

1 cup onion, diced

1 cup carrots, diced

1 cup diced Idaho potatoes

2 garlic cloves, minced

2 bay leaves

1 teaspoon all-natural sea salt

1 teaspoon freshly ground black pepper

1 cup plain nonfat yogurt

1. In a slow cooker, combine the water, peas, celery, onion, carrots, potatoes, minced garlic, bay leaves, sea salt, and pepper.

2. Set the slow cooker to low for 8–9 hours.

3. Remove from heat and allow to cool.

4. Slowly stir in the yogurt until well-blended.

PER SERVING Calories: 107.54 | Fat: 1.70 g | Protein: 5.27 g | Sodium: 467.54 mg | Fiber: 4.78 g | Carbohydrates: 18.65 g | Sugar: 7.67 g

No Fat Needed

Lean meats are not only acceptable for a clean lifestyle, they're highly recommended. When it comes to what constitutes a lean meat, though, things can get tricky. It's true that ham is a cut of pork, but the difference from a pork tenderloin isn't just the area of the pig it comes from, but the fat content between the two cuts of meat. The same concept applies to beef when you compare a beef tenderloin and a rib eye. When you're shopping for meats, just make sure that the flavor you'll be enjoying will come from the meat itself, and not its fat.

Chicken Fajita Soup

Sure, fajitas aren't normally thought of in soup form! This recipe will change your mind about that. Enjoy all your favorite fajita flavors in a different format.

INGREDIENTS | SERVES 4

3 cups filtered water

1 tablespoon minced garlic

1 red pepper, sliced

1 yellow pepper, sliced

1 poblano pepper, sliced

1 large yellow onion, sliced

3 boneless, skinless chicken breasts, cut into bite-sized pieces

2 cups plain nonfat yogurt

1 teaspoon all-natural sea salt

1 teaspoon freshly ground black pepper

2 teaspoons cayenne pepper

3 tablespoons cumin powder

1. In a large pot over medium heat, combine the water and garlic, and bring to a boil. Reduce heat to low and simmer for 5 minutes.

2. Add the peppers and onions to the pot and simmer for 8–10 minutes.

3. Add the chicken to the pot and simmer for 5–8 minutes, or until chicken is cooked through.

4. Remove from heat and cool for about 5 minutes.

5. Stir in the yogurt and spices, and blend well.

PER SERVING Calories: 226.30 | Fat: 7.93 g | Protein: 24.34 g | Sodium: 728.12 mg | Fiber: 2.55 g | Carbohydrates: 15.57 g | Sugar: 9.12 g

Chicken Noodle

This classic soup is a great way to treat a cold or warm up on a chilly day. Appealing to kids of all ages, this is one classic dish made clean!

INGREDIENTS | SERVES 4

1 tablespoon olive oil

1 tablespoon minced garlic

2 cups chopped yellow onion

2 cups chopped celery

2 cups chopped carrots

1 tablespoon dried basil

1 tablespoon dried tarragon

1 tablespoon dried thyme

2 teaspoons all-natural sea salt

4 cups filtered water

3 boneless, skinless chicken breasts, cut into bite-sized pieces

1 cup 100% whole wheat pasta shells

1. In a large pot over medium heat, sauté the olive oil, garlic, onions, celery, and carrots with the spices for 7–10 minutes or until tender. Reduce heat to low.

2. Add the water, and simmer for about 20 minutes.

3. Add chicken and continue to simmer for about 10 minutes, or until chicken is cooked through.

4. Add the pasta, stirring constantly, and simmer until pasta is al dente.

5. Remove from heat and serve.

PER SERVING Calories: 270.26 | Fat: 6.78 g | Protein: 22.9 g | Sodium: 1342.57 mg | Fiber: 6.64 g | Carbohydrates: 30.75 g | Sugar: 7.53 g

use lots of chicken broth

Tips to Clean Up the Traditional

When it comes to some of your favorite traditional soups, the classic recipes may have a little more fat, calories, and sodium than you expected. That's where clean eating comes to the rescue! Taking chicken noodle soup, for example, you would make it clean by seasoning and softening the vegetables in extra-virgin olive oil (rather than butter) and spices before adding the water; this one step would heighten the flavors of the spices, perfectly sauté the veggies, and make for a delicious broth background for your soup. Using chicken breast instead of dark meat and whole wheat pasta instead of refined are just two more healthy substitutes that improve the nutritional content while maintaining great taste.

Turkey with Meatballs

These delicious sausage-like homemade turkey meatballs are mouthwatering, and with all of the natural ingredients that promote amazing health benefits in such a tasty dish, how could anyone resist the temptation to live the clean life?

INGREDIENTS | SERVES 6

4 cups filtered water

2 cups Tasty Tomato Sauce (see recipe in Chapter 4)

1 tablespoon minced garlic

1 cup onion, chopped

2 cups celery, chopped

2 cups Idaho potatoes, chopped

2 cups carrots, chopped

½ pound ground organic turkey breast

1 egg

1 slice sprouted grain bread, crumbled

1 tablespoon coriander seeds

1 teaspoon garlic powder

1 teaspoon onion powder

1 teaspoon all-natural sea salt

1 teaspoon freshly ground black pepper

2 cups cooked 100% whole wheat pasta ribbons

1. In a large pot over medium heat, bring the water, tomato sauce, garlic, onion, celery, potatoes, and carrots to a boil. Reduce heat to low, and simmer for 20–30 minutes.

2. In a mixing bowl, combine the turkey breast, egg, breadcrumbs, coriander seeds, garlic powder, and onion powder, and blend well. Roll the mixture into mini meatballs.

3. Place the meatballs in the soup and continue to simmer for another 20 minutes or until meatballs are cooked through. Remove from heat.

4. Season with salt and pepper to taste, and serve over pasta.

PER SERVING Calories: 252.73 | Fat: 2.09 g | Protein: 17.63 g | Sodium: 954.56 mg | Fiber: 8.00 g | Carbohydrates: 43.36 g | Sugar: 8.43 g

Go Extreme for Big Flavor

Soups that use lean meats have intense flavors from the additional spices and combinations used to prepare them. Whipping up a batch of low-fat meatballs that contain coriander seeds with a bite is an extra step, but one that adds flavor, texture, and a delicious unexpected element that would leave the soup rather boring if left out.

Cream of Mushroom Soup

The traditional version of this beloved comfort food is loaded with cream, milk, and loads of salt. By cleaning up this warm, earthy soup, you can enjoy it anytime . . . guilt-free!

INGREDIENTS | SERVES 4

5 cups unsweetened almond milk

1 large white potato, peeled and diced

1 cup white onion, diced

1 cup chopped baby portabella mushrooms

1 cup chopped cremini mushrooms

1 cup chopped oyster mushrooms

2 tablespoons minced garlic

1 cup plain low-fat Greek style yogurt

2 teaspoons all-natural sea salt

2 teaspoons freshly ground black pepper

1. In a large saucepan, combine the almond milk, potato, onion, and minced garlic over medium heat, and bring to a simmer for 15 minutes or until all contents are tender.

2. Using an immersion blender, emulsify the potato and onion until completely blended and no chunks remain.

3. Continuing over medium heat, add the mushrooms to the saucepan and simmer until all mushrooms are soft, about 15 minutes.

4. Remove the saucepan from the heat, add the yogurt, salt, and pepper, and, using the immersion blender, emulsify the mushrooms into the soup until only small bits of mushrooms remain.

PER SERVING Calories: 302.593 | Fat: 6.595 g | Protein: 16.709 g | Sodium: 1390.409 mg | Fiber: 5.769 g | Carbohydrates: 45.65 g | Sugar: 20.152 g

Meaty Black Bean Stew

The healthy ingredients used throughout this recipe make this a not guilty pleasure you can enjoy anytime. It's an amazing combination of hearty vegetables.

INGREDIENTS | SERVES 6

½ pound ground lean beef

1 tablespoon minced garlic

1 yellow onion, minced

3 cups Tasty Tomato Sauce (see recipe in Chapter 4)

3 cups filtered water

2 teaspoons cumin

2 teaspoons chili powder

2 cups kernel corn

4 cups black beans, soaked and drained

2 large tomatoes, chopped

1. In a large pot over medium heat, brown the beef, minced garlic, and yellow onion together until beef is cooked through and onion is tender.

2. Drain the extra fat, return the pot to the heat, and add the tomato sauce, water, and spices. Bring to a simmer, then reduce heat to low.

3. Add the corn and half of the beans to the pot, and continue to simmer for about 15 minutes.

4. In a blender or food processor, combine the remaining black beans and the tomatoes, purée, and add to the soup pot.

5. Mix the soup well until thoroughly blended, and continue to simmer for about 10 minutes.

6. Serve hot or cold.

PER SERVING Calories: 305.77 | Fat: 4.70 g | Protein: 21.10 g | Sodium: 1186.08 mg | Fiber: 13.60 g | Carbohydrates: 48.72 g | Sugar: 12.38 g

Tortilla Soup

This recipe is a festive collection of amazing fresh vegetables that complement one another perfectly. Mild tomatoes and sweet corn balance the spicy green chilies, onions, and tantalizing spices, resulting in a great-tasting dish the whole family will enjoy.

INGREDIENTS | SERVES 4

2 cups filtered water

2 cups Tasty Tomato Sauce (see recipe in Chapter 4)

2 cups cooked boneless, skinless chicken breast, torn

2 cups chopped tomatoes

2 cups frozen corn

1 yellow onion, chopped

½ cup green chilies, chopped

1 tablespoon chili powder

1 tablespoon cumin

2 teaspoons garlic powder

2 teaspoons onion powder

1 teaspoon all-natural sea salt

1 teaspoon freshly ground black pepper

1. In a slow cooker, combine all of the ingredients and mix well.

2. Set the slow cooker to low for 8–9 hours.

3. Serve with Tasty Tortilla Chips (see recipe in Chapter 4).

PER SERVING Calories: 293.57 | Fat: 4.70 g | Protein: 30.46 g | Sodium: 1388.20 mg | Fiber: 7.20 g | Carbohydrates: 37.69 g | Sugar: 13.08 g

Creamy Corn Chowder

Most people don't think of chowder as being the healthiest or most calorie-conscious of meal options, but this recipe breaks the mold. It's packed with delicious, all-natural ingredients specifically chosen for their nutrition and taste.

INGREDIENTS | SERVES 6

6 cups almond milk, divided
1 cup potatoes, peeled and chopped
1 cup carrots, chopped
4 cups kernel corn
1 teaspoon all-natural sea salt
1 cup low-fat plain Greek-style yogurt

1. In a large pot over medium heat, bring 3 cups of the almond milk, potatoes, and carrots to a boil. Reduce heat to low and simmer for 10 minutes.

2. Add remaining 3 cups almond milk, kernel corn, and salt, and simmer for another 5–8 minutes.

3. Remove the soup from the heat and allow to cool about 5 minutes.

4. Slowly mix in ¼ cup of the Greek yogurt at a time until well blended.

PER SERVING Calories: 115.98 | Fat: 0.28 g | Protein: 6.86 g | Sodium: 607.99 mg | Fiber: 2.88 g | Carbohydrates: 13.80 g | Sugar: 3.83 g

CHAPTER 12

Refreshing Salads

Spicy Eggs with Romaine and Arugula

Hard-boiled eggs sprinkled with tasty spices provide a protein-rich topping on this crisp salad. These flavors are the perfect answer if your salads have gotten boring!

INGREDIENTS | SERVES 2

2 tablespoons red wine vinegar
1 tablespoon extra-virgin olive oil
1 teaspoon all-natural sea salt
1 teaspoon freshly ground black pepper
1½ cups romaine lettuce, chopped
1½ cups arugula, chopped
4 hard-boiled eggs, peeled
1 teaspoon cayenne pepper

Protein-Packed Salads

If you try to incorporate complex carbs, lean proteins, and healthy fats at every meal, you'll see just how versatile salads can be. Topping crunchy lettuce of any type (complex carbohydrate) with eggs, lean chicken, beef, or fish (protein), and tossing it with extra-virgin olive oil (healthy fat) creates a food combination of every important element your body needs.

1. In a mixing bowl, whisk together the red wine vinegar, olive oil, sea salt, and pepper until well blended.

2. In the vinegar and olive oil, toss the lettuces to coat.

3. Halve the eggs and sprinkle the cayenne evenly atop each of the 8 halves.

4. Serve half of the dressed salad in each of two bowls, and top with the egg halves.

PER SERVING Calories: 220.78 | Fat: 17.08 g | Protein: 13.62 g | Sodium: 1327.82 mg | Fiber: 1.50 g | Carbohydrates: 3.72 g | Sugar: 1.59 g

Asparagus Spears and Grape Tomato Toss

Blanched asparagus spears add a beautiful bright green to this delicious toss, while the grape tomatoes contribute a deep red. It's a feast for your eyes and your taste buds.

INGREDIENTS | SERVES 2

4 cups asparagus spears, cut into 1" strips

2 cups grape tomatoes, halved

2 tablespoons balsamic vinegar

1 tablespoon extra-virgin olive oil

Don't Diet, Eat Clean!

If you're fed up with diets, clean eating is a great lifestyle to adopt. With clean eating, you'll eat more frequently, so you'll feel less hungry. The foods available in the clean lifestyle are just as tasty and satisfying, but they're made with clean, healthy ingredients that all contribute something to your body's functioning. The combining of foods for optimum nutrition is one of the most appealing attributes because you never feel tired, run down, or sluggish.

1. In a pot of boiling water over medium heat, blanch the asparagus spears for less than 1 minute, until bright green and still crisp. Remove from heat and shock with cold water to stop the cooking process.

2. Remove the asparagus from the pot and place in a mixing bowl.

3. Add the halved grape tomatoes to the mixing bowl, and drizzle the balsamic and olive oil over the salad.

4. Toss to coat evenly, and serve in two salad bowls.

PER SERVING Calories: 154.12 | Fat: 7.37 g | Protein: 7.29 g | Sodium: 16.61 mg | Fiber: 7.42 g | Carbohydrates: 18.96 g | Sugar: 11.34 g

Grilled Tomato and Pesto Salad

A fresh tomato salad is always tasty—but this version takes things up a notch by grilling some of the ingredients. Give it a try as an appetizer at your next barbecue!

INGREDIENTS | SERVES 2

2 large beefsteak tomatoes, sliced in ¼" slices

1 cup prepared Peppy Pesto (see recipe in Chapter 4)

2 cups romaine lettuce, chopped

Cravings Decoded

Sometimes the body craves certain foods because it needs something that the food provides. Cheeseburger cravings may indicate a protein deficiency, just as a sudden hankering for chips may be a need for complex carbohydrates. Rather than listening to your exact cravings, instead try to figure out what your body may *really* be telling you it needs. Then give it what it wants, in a clean way!

1. Prepare a grill with olive oil spray over medium heat.

2. Paint the tomato slices on just one side with the Peppy Pesto.

3. Set the pesto-painted sides of the tomatoes face-down on the grill, and paint the other side with the Peppy Pesto also.

4. Grill each side for about 2–3 minutes, and remove from heat.

5. In two salad bowls, with 1 cup of the chopped romaine in each, evenly divide the grilled tomatoes, and serve.

PER SERVING Calories: 395.42 | Fat: 34.11 g | Protein: 9.65 g | Sodium: 684.86 mg | Fiber: 3.17 g | Carbohydrates: 12.41 g | Sugar: 5.35 g

Simple Spinach Salad

Baby spinach leaves are so tasty on their own, they really need little else to be the perfect salad. Adding cool cucumber and crisp sunflower seeds in a light coating of extra-virgin olive oil and balsamic vinegar brings out the best in this dish.

INGREDIENTS | SERVES 2

1 tablespoon balsamic vinegar

1 tablespoon extra-virgin olive oil

2 cups baby spinach leaves, washed

1 cucumber, peeled and sliced

2 tablespoons toasted, unsalted sunflower seeds

1. In a large mixing bowl, whisk together the balsamic vinegar and olive oil.

2. Add the spinach leaves to the mixing bowl, and toss to coat.

3. Split the spinach salad between two bowls, and top with cucumbers and sunflower seeds.

PER SERVING Calories: 148.72 | Fat: 11.66 g | Protein: 3.75 g | Sodium: 29.49 g | Fiber: 2.19 g | Carbohydrates: 9.71 g | Sugar: 4.07 g

Sweetened Spinach Salad

Spinach leaves bring something extra to a salad: iron. It's easy to get part of your daily recommended allowance with this salad!

INGREDIENTS | SERVES 2

1 tablespoon red wine vinegar

1 tablespoon extra-virgin olive oil

1 tablespoon ground flaxseed

½ tablespoon agave nectar

2 cups baby spinach, washed

½ English cucumber, halved and sliced

1 cup dried, unsweetened cranberries

2 tablespoons toasted, unsalted pine nuts

1. In a large mixing bowl, whisk together the vinegar, olive oil, flaxseed, and agave until well blended.

2. Toss the spinach leaves in the dressing, and split the salad between two salad bowls.

3. Top the salads with the cucumbers, dried cranberries, and pine nuts.

PER SERVING Calories: 300.52 | Fat: 25.30 g | Protein: 5.18 g | Sodium: 45.80 mg | Fiber: 7.12 g | Carbohydrates: 18.13 g | Sugar: 6.50 g

Bean and Couscous Craziness

Packed with nutrition, this salad is a great way to serve up couscous. No longer a boring, bland side dish, this salad recipe jazzes up couscous with protein-packed white beans, scallions with a bite, and sweet peas.

INGREDIENTS | SERVES 2

2 cups prepared couscous

1 cup white beans, soaked and drained

¼ cup scallions, chopped

¼ cup sweet peas

2 tablespoons balsamic vinegar

1 tablespoon extra-virgin olive oil

1. In a large mixing bowl, combine the couscous, beans, scallions, and peas, and blend thoroughly.

2. Add the balsamic and olive oil over the mix, and toss to coat, combining well.

3. Serve hot or cold.

PER SERVING Calories: 1042.92 | Fat: 8.6 g | Protein: 42.35 g | Sodium: 39.83 mg | Fiber: 26.7 g | Carbohydrates: 196.38 g | Sugar: 11.57 g

What's Your Salad?

There's absolutely no reason why a salad has to be lettuce, tomato, and cucumber. When you start getting creative and figuring out exactly what it is you love about salads, you'll start craving them like any other favorite food. Maybe salty ingredients like olives, artichokes, and roasted red peppers call your name, or the sweet and crunchy combination of dried fruit and nuts does the trick. Whatever the case may be, you can figure out a great salad that does your body good and does your taste buds great!

Spinach, Tomato, and Mozzarella

This light and delicious combination of baby spinach leaves, light tomato slices, and melt-in-your-mouth mozzarella slices is as beautiful as it is tasty. Add dried basil leaves in a drizzle of olive oil, and you're in heaven!

INGREDIENTS | SERVES 2

2 cups baby spinach leaves, washed

1 cup tomatoes, chopped

½ cup fresh buffalo mozzarella, chopped

2 tablespoons extra-virgin olive oil

2 teaspoons dried basil leaves

1. Set out two salad bowls, and split the spinach evenly between the two.

2. Top each salad with half of the tomatoes.

3. Top each salad with half of the mozzarella.

4. Drizzle the olive oil over the top of both salads and sprinkle with the dried basil.

PER SERVING Calories: 226.64 | Fat: 20.06 g | Protein: 7.89 g | Sodium: 204.07 mg | Fiber: 1.75 g | Carbohydrates: 5.25 g | Sugar: 2.78 g

Asian Almond Mandarin

You sometimes see salads like this at restaurants. Using simple vinegars that contain little or no calories, fat, sugar, or sodium in combination with healthy sesame oil, natural agave nectar, and powerful ginger makes for a tasty dish with little or no additives!

INGREDIENTS | SERVES 2

1 tablespoon rice wine vinegar

1 tablespoon sesame oil

1 teaspoon agave nectar

1 tablespoon fresh ginger, minced

2 cups endive leaves, chopped

½ cup slivered almonds

1 cup mandarin oranges slices

1. In a mixing bowl, whisk together the vinegar, sesame oil, agave, and the minced ginger until well blended.

2. Toss the chopped endive leaves in the dressing to coat.

3. Split the salad between two salad bowls.

4. Top evenly with the slivered almonds and mandarin oranges.

PER SERVING Calories: 283.75 | Fat: 19.09 g | Protein: 6.90 g | Sodium: 5.59 mg | Fiber: 7.79 g | Carbohydrates: 26.59 g | Sugar: 14.23 g

Spicy Black Bean Tex-Mex Salad

Crisp, cool romaine gets all spiced up with a delicious blend of black beans, sweet corn, and chopped tomatoes in a spicy sauce. Olive oil lightly dresses the combination, but makes sure the spicy cayenne and aromatic cumin stick!

INGREDIENTS | SERVES 2

1 tablespoon extra-virgin olive oil

1 cup black beans, soaked and drained

1 cup corn kernels

1 cup chopped tomatoes

1 teaspoon cayenne pepper

1 teaspoon cumin

2 cups romaine lettuce, chopped

Any Meal Can Be a Salad

If you start getting really creative with your salads, you can start converting your favorite dishes into healthier versions. Take any cuisine like Asian, Italian, Mediterranean, Southern, or Mexican, and you can twist any favorite recipe into a salad recipe. Start with a bed of lettuce, and start loading up the ingredients. Whether the spices are what make the cuisine unique, or the protein sources that make it great, throw them in a salad.

1. In a large mixing bowl, combine the olive oil, black beans, corn, and tomatoes with the cayenne and cumin, and toss to coat.

2. Add the chopped romaine lettuce, and toss to thoroughly combine.

3. Divide the salad evenly between two salad bowls, and serve.

PER SERVING Calories: 275.49 | Fat: 8.70 g | Protein: 10.92 g | Sodium: 393.05 mg | Fiber: 11.25 g | Carbohydrates: 43.35 g | Sugar: 8.42 g

Strawberry Walnut Flaxseed Salad

No need for lettuce here! There's plenty of filling ingredients in this wonderful salad already.

INGREDIENTS | SERVES 2

4 cups strawberries, tops removed
1 cup walnuts, crushed
2 tablespoons ground flaxseed
1 tablespoon red wine vinegar
½ tablespoon agave nectar
2 sprigs mint leaves

Sneak Your Nutrition into Every Bite

Adding a beautiful appearance, a nutty flavor, and a delicious crunch to your salads, flaxseeds also contribute essential fats without any effort at all.

1. Quarter the strawberries and place in a mixing bowl.

2. Add the walnuts and ground flaxseed to the strawberries.

3. Drizzle the red wine vinegar and agave over the salad, and toss to coat.

4. Split the salad between two salad bowls, garnish each with a mint sprig, and serve.

PER SERVING Calories: 516.15 | Fat: 41.61 g | Protein: 12.58 g | Sodium: 4.72 mg | Fiber: 11.99 g | Carbohydrates: 33.92 g | Sugar: 17.06

Chicken and Apple Spinach Salad

This recipe is a great way to use up some leftover grilled chicken breast. The Granny Smith apple offers a refreshing crunch.

INGREDIENTS | SERVES 2

1 Granny Smith apple, cored and chopped
1 cup cooked boneless, skinless chicken breast, torn into bite-sized pieces
½ cup crushed walnuts
2 cups nonfat vanilla yogurt
1 tablespoon agave nectar
2 cups baby spinach, washed

1. In a large mixing bowl, combine the apples, chicken, and walnuts with the nonfat yogurt and agave.

2. After blending well, add the spinach to the bowl and toss to coat.

3. Divide the salad evenly between two salad bowls, and serve.

PER SERVING Calories: 546.17 | Fat: 30.16 g | Protein: 37.84 g | Sodium: 267.33 mg | Fiber: 3.69 g | Carbohydrates: 35.52 g | Sugar: 29.14 g

Tuna-Topped Salad

This delicious tuna recipe makes for a great standalone dish, so just imagine how tasty it is served atop crisp romaine lettuce. Tasty, and beautifully served, this is a delicious dish you can be proud to serve up to family or friends. It's time to think outside the (tuna) can!

INGREDIENTS | SERVES 2

1 teaspoon low-sodium soy sauce

1 tablespoon minced garlic

2 tablespoons freshly minced ginger

2 tablespoons rice wine vinegar

2 tuna steaks

1 tablespoon canola oil

3 cups chopped romaine lettuce

1 tablespoon sesame oil

½ cup scallions, chopped

1. In a shallow dish, combine the soy sauce, minced garlic, 1 tablespoon of the ginger, and 1 tablespoon of the rice wine vinegar and set the tuna steaks in the marinade. Refrigerate for 30 minutes, turning once after 15 minutes.

2. Prepare a large skillet with the canola oil over medium heat and place the tuna steaks in the skillet.

3. Sauté the tuna steaks for 4–6 minutes on each side, or until the tuna is completely cooked through.

4. In a mixing bowl, combine the chopped romaine with the sesame oil and remaining ginger and rice wine vinegar, and toss to coat.

5. Split the dressed lettuce between two salad bowls, top with the tuna steaks, and garnish with the chopped scallions.

PER SERVING Calories: 489.27 | Fat: 25.26 g | Protein: 54.13 g | Sodium: 100.25 mg | Fiber: 2.68 g | Carbohydrates: 8.97 g | Sugar: 2.25 g

Fruit Salad with Ginger and Lemon Juice

Traditional fruit salad is just a few fruits and melons thrown together and served. This recipe includes a tasty dressing of freshly squeezed lemon juice and minced ginger for a heightened flavor experience that will make fruit salad mean something completely new.

INGREDIENTS | SERVES 4

1 grapefruit, inside pieces removed

1 cup pineapple chunks

1 cup green seedless grapes, sliced

1 Granny Smith apple, cored, sliced, and chopped

1 cup cubed cantaloupe

1 cup cubed honeydew melon

3 tablespoons freshly squeezed lemon juice

2 tablespoons freshly grated ginger

1. In a mixing bowl, combine the fruit, lemon juice, and grated ginger.

2. Toss to coat and combine thoroughly and share between two salad bowls.

PER SERVING Calories: 126.80 | Fat: 0.55 g | Protein: 1.86 g | Sodium: 18.32 mg | Fiber: 3.22 g | Carbohydrates: 32.25 g | Sugar: 25.32 g

Citrus to Brighten Fruit Flavors

Most fruit salads are delicious just as they are, and it's pretty difficult to create a bad-tasting combination of sweet fruits. Heightening and brightening the flavors, though, is easily done with just a simple addition of citrus juice. Even if you don't particularly like lemon juice or lime juice on its own, you may find that it is the perfect addition to your fruit salads because of its amazing ability to brighten the colors and the flavors of the fruit. Just as the addition of salt to sweet cookie mix sounds contradictory but works, tart lemon juice works wonders for fruit.

Thai Beef Strip Salad

This is a great salad that's packed with marinated steak, fresh ingredients, and delicious, aromatic spices. Unique and definitely different from the usual dinner salad, this is a great appetizer, side, or main dish. You'll love the tender steak, crisp veggies, and delicious dressing.

INGREDIENTS | SERVES 4

2 cups lime juice

½ cup fish sauce

1 cucumber, peeled and sliced

1 pint cherry tomatoes, washed

½ cup mint, chopped

½ cup cilantro, chopped

1 cup scallions, chopped

1 cup lemongrass, in 1" chunks

1 pound flank steak

6 cups romaine lettuce, chopped

Steak Lovers Rejoice!

Clean eating never tasted so good! If you're a steak lover, you will be happy to hear that lean steak strips atop a beautiful combination of vegetables is one of the healthiest meals you can eat. By combining the beautiful strips of steak cooked to whatever doneness you desire, and delicious, fresh vegetables like lettuce and whatever else you think will be a tasty side-kick to your steak, you have a complex carbohydrate, protein, and healthy fat combination that constitutes the perfect meal.

1. Prepare a grill to medium heat and spray with olive oil spray.

2. In a large mixing bowl, combine the lime juice, fish sauce, cucumber slices, tomatoes, mint, cilantro, scallions, and lemongrass, and mix together until well combined.

3. Paint one side of the steak with the marinade, and place on the grill for about 7 minutes. Paint the unseasoned side and flip the steak to continue cooking for another 7 minutes or until cooked through.

4. Remove the steak from the grill, and allow to cool for about 10 minutes before slicing thinly (about ¼"–½"). Place steak slices in the marinade and allow to soak for 1 hour or more.

5. In a large salad bowl, toss the chopped romaine, marinated steak, and vegetable combination to coat completely.

PER SERVING Calories: 235.22 | Fat: 8.78 g | Protein: 26.65 g | Sodium: 2307.29 mg | Fiber: 4.14 g | Carbohydrates: 11.01 g | Sugar: 5.24 g

Sweet and Spicy Shrimp Salad

Light cooked shrimp gets all dressed up in a sweet and spicy sauce of agave nectar and red pepper flakes to make for an interesting and delicious twist to any plain salad. Crisp romaine makes for the perfect crunch to accompany the tasty, tender shrimp with sweetness and spice!

INGREDIENTS | SERVES 2

1 tablespoon extra-virgin olive oil

1 tablespoon red wine vinegar

1 tablespoon agave nectar

½ tablespoon red pepper flakes

¼ pound cooked medium shrimp, peeled and chilled

2 cups romaine lettuce, chopped

1. In a large mixing bowl, combine the olive oil, vinegar, agave, and red pepper flakes.

2. Toss the shrimp in the sauce to coat.

3. Add the chopped romaine to the mixing bowl, and toss to coat.

4. Share the salad between two salad bowls, and serve.

PER SERVING Calories: 164.86 | Fat: 8.09 g | Protein: 12.15 g | Sodium: 88.19 mg | Fiber: 1.37 g | Carbohydrates: 11.56 g | Sugar: 9.40 g

Creamy Macaroni Salad

That macaroni salad that calls your name at every summer party gets a clean makeover with this recipe. Delicious, nutritious, and absolutely beautiful, this salad has a mayo-esque flavor with none of the guilt!

INGREDIENTS | SERVES 4

2 cups plain nonfat yogurt

1 tablespoon white vinegar

2 cups cooked 100% whole wheat elbow macaroni pasta

1 cup sweet petite peas

1 cup chopped red pepper

1 cup chopped yellow pepper

1. In a small dish, combine the yogurt and vinegar well.

2. Add the cooked pasta to the yogurt and toss to coat.

3. Stir the peas, red pepper, and yellow pepper into the creamy pasta.

4. Refrigerate at least one hour, but best overnight.

PER SERVING Calories: 457.39 | Fat: 9.08 g | Protein: 24.81 g | Sodium: 74.49 mg | Fiber: 23.76 g | Carbohydrates: 78.77 g | Sugar: 13.54 g

Salad Niçoise

Here's this hearty tuna salad, all cleaned up. The tangy dressing will surprise you!

INGREDIENTS | SERVES 2

3 tablespoons olive oil

1 tablespoon white vinegar

1 teaspoon dried mustard

1 can solid white albacore tuna in water, drained

4 medium tomatoes, wedged

2 cups cooked Idaho potatoes, cubed and boiled

1 cup blanched green beans, trimmed

½ cup sliced black or green olives

2 tablespoons capers, rinsed

1. In a large mixing bowl, whisk together the olive oil, vinegar, and mustard.

2. Add the tuna, tomato wedges, boiled potatoes, green beans, olives, and capers.

3. Blend ingredients well.

4. Share the salad evenly between two salad bowls, and serve.

PER SERVING Calories: 556.83 | Fat: 31.80 g | Protein: 31.20 g | Sodium: 905.28 mg | Fiber: 9.46 g | Carbohydrates: 39.71 g | Sugar: 10.05 g

Try New Things

Just like children, sometimes adults think they know what they like and what they don't, and they don't deviate from their tastes. However, you may be pleasantly surprised when you try something you were adamantly convinced you would hate. So just like you tell your kids—*try* it and see if you like it!

Macaroni Salad with Sautéed Veggies and Vinaigrette

This carbohydrate-loaded pasta salad uses all clean ingredients to deliver health on a platter.

INGREDIENTS | SERVES 4

1 cup yellow pepper slices

1 cup red pepper slices

1 cup yellow onion slices

1 tablespoon olive oil

1 teaspoon all-natural sea salt

2 tablespoons balsamic vinegar

2 cups cooked 100% whole wheat rigatoni

Bell Peppers for Better Health

With almost 300 percent of the daily recommended value of vitamin C, yellow and orange peppers can lend health benefits and a delightfully fruity taste to any dish.

1. In a large skillet over medium heat, sauté the sliced vegetables with the olive oil and sea salt until tender, about 5 minutes.

2. Remove the peppers and onions from the heat and allow to cool.

3. In a large mixing bowl, combine the chopped romaine, tossed veggies, and balsamic until thoroughly combined.

PER SERVING Calories: 206.93 | Fat: 4.34 g | Protein: 6.72 g | Sodium: 598.38 mg | Fiber: 6.75 g | Carbohydrates: 38.15 g | Sugar: 5.47 g

Cucumber Salad

Two varieties of cool, crisp cucumbers get all shaken up in this delicious salad.
Bring it to your next party or potluck and know it'll be a hit!

INGREDIENTS | SERVES 2

1 tablespoon olive oil

1 teaspoon garlic powder

1 tablespoon red wine vinegar

2 tablespoons minced dill

½ cup plain nonfat yogurt

1 English cucumber, sliced

1 cucumber, peeled and sliced

½ cup sliced Vidalia onion

1. In a large mixing bowl, whisk the olive oil, garlic powder, vinegar, dill, and yogurt together until well combined.

2. Fold in the sliced cucumbers and onions, and toss to coat.

3. Share between two salad bowls, and serve.

PER SERVING Calories: 148.48 | Fat: 9.10 g | Protein: 4.34 g | Sodium: 36.11 mg | Fiber: 1.64 g | Carbohydrates: 14.86 g | Sugar: 7.92 g

Endive and Avocado

Spicy bites from the olives and vinegar get balanced beautifully with the refreshing flavors and textures of fresh tomato, avocado, and mozzarella cheese for an amazing salad that looks great, tastes great, and does wonders for your boring lunchtime routine!

INGREDIENTS | SERVES 2

2 tablespoons extra-virgin olive oil
1 tablespoon red wine vinegar
1 teaspoon all-natural sea salt
1 teaspoon freshly ground black pepper
2 tomatoes, wedged
½ cup black olives, sliced
2 cups whole endive leaves
1 cup fresh buffalo mozzarella, sliced
1 avocado, peeled and sliced

1. In a large mixing bowl, combine the olive oil, vinegar, sea salt, pepper, tomatoes, and olives, and toss to coat.

2. Set the endive leaves evenly between two salad bowls, and cover with the tossed oil, vinegar, and vegetable combination.

3. Top the salads with the mozzarella slices, and garnish with the slices of avocado.

PER SERVING Calories: 467.58 | Fat: 40.87 g | Protein: 15.36 g | Sodium: 1540.18 mg | Fiber: 9.81 g | Carbohydrates: 14.11 g | Sugar: 1.25 g

"Cool as a Cucumber" Tabbouleh Salad

This is an incredibly versatile dish that can be eaten alone, wrapped in a tortilla, stuffed in a pita, or even used as a delicious topping for rice, pasta, or quinoa!

INGREDIENTS | SERVES 2

2 large cucumbers, peeled and chopped
2 tablespoons extra-virgin olive oil
2 tablespoons red wine vinegar
2 cups cooked bulgur

1. Combine the cucumbers, olive oil, and vinegar in a mixing bowl, and toss to combine.

2. Fold the bulgur into the cucumber mix, and combine thoroughly.

3. Refrigerate for 1 hour, and serve in two salad bowls.

PER SERVING Calories: 279.33 | Fat: 17.83 g | Protein: 4.96 g | Sodium: 44.28 mg | Fiber: 5.31 g | Carbohydrates: 28.37 g | Sugar: 5.03 g

Cucumbers for . . . Everything

Not only are cucumbers heralded for their high water content, they are also packed with an amazing nutrient called silica, which may make your skin look and feel younger, your nails stronger, and your hair shinier.

Tomato Caprese Salad

This Italian favorite is so simple, and yet so amazingly delicious! Going out to an expensive restaurant is no longer necessary. By yourself, or loaded up with guests, you can feel precious and pampered with this light, healthy, satisfying salad!

INGREDIENTS | SERVES 2

4 large tomatoes, sliced
2 tablespoons extra-virgin olive oil
1 teaspoon all-natural sea salt
1 teaspoon freshly ground black pepper
½ cup basil leaves
1 cup fresh buffalo mozzarella, sliced

1. Layer the tomatoes evenly on two plates, drizzle with the olive oil, and sprinkle with the salt and pepper.

2. Top the tomatoes with the basil leaves.

3. Layer the mozzarella over the tomatoes and basil, and serve.

PER SERVING Calories: 336.78 | Fat: 26.61 g | Protein: 15.03 g | Sodium: 1543.47 mg | Fiber: 3.40 g | Carbohydrates: 11.84 g | Sugar: 7.09 g

Classic Antipasto

Forget ordering this delicious dish from a restaurant that uses ingredients of questionable quality. Normally loaded with huge amounts of sodium and empty calories, this lightened-up version keeps it clean!

INGREDIENTS | SERVES 4

2 cups black olives
2 cups artichoke hearts
2 cups roasted red pepper strips
8 pepperoncinis
1 cup banana peppers
4 tablespoons white vinegar
4 cups chopped romaine
2 tablespoons red wine vinegar
2 tablespoons olive oil
1 tablespoon dried oregano

1. In a large shallow dish, combine the olives, artichokes, red peppers, pepperoncinis, and banana peppers in the white vinegar. Soak for 1 hour, tossing consistently.

2. In a large mixing bowl, combine the romaine, red wine vinegar, olive oil, and oregano, and toss to coat.

3. Drain the vegetables, and add them to the romaine. Toss to blend thoroughly.

PER SERVING Calories: 288.01 | Fat: 15.16 g | Protein: 10.28 g | Sodium: 1276.97 mg | Fiber: 21.92 g | Carbohydrates: 43.69 g | Sugar: 6.82 g

Chilled Steak Salad

Taking a delicious flank steak, grilling it, and infusing it with the amazing flavors of balsamic vinegar, garlic, salt, and pepper is a great idea. An even better twist on that great idea is to slice it and use it as a delicious topping on a beautiful crisp, simple salad of romaine and tomato.

INGREDIENTS | SERVES 4

1 pound flank steak
2 tablespoons balsamic vinegar
1 teaspoon all-natural sea salt
2 teaspoons garlic powder
1 teaspoon freshly ground black pepper
4 cups romaine lettuce, chopped
1 large tomato, wedged into 8 pieces
1 tablespoon extra-virgin olive oil
1 cup crumbled goat cheese

1. Prepare a grill over medium heat with olive oil spray, and set the steak on the grill grate.

2. Drizzle the steak with ½ tablespoon of balsamic vinegar and a light sprinkling of the salt, garlic powder, and pepper. Grill for about 5–8 minutes, and flip.

3. Drizzle the other ½ tablespoon of balsamic over the steak with the remaining salt, garlic powder, and pepper, and grill for 5–8 minutes, or until cooked through.

4. Remove the steak from the grill, and allow to cool. Slice thinly.

5. In a mixing bowl, toss the chopped romaine and tomato wedges with the tablespoon of balsamic vinegar and olive oil, and share between two salad bowls.

6. Top the salads with the steak and finish with the crumbled goat cheese, and serve.

PER SERVING Calories: 475.10 | Fat: 31.43 g | Protein: 41.46 g | Sodium: 848.20 mg | Fiber: 0.64 g | Carbohydrates: 5.14 g | Sugar: 3.25 g

Delectable Desserts

Clean Whipped Cream

This is a great clean version of the typically fat-laden whipped topping. With only three delicious ingredients whipped together for a delightfully light and sweet treat, this is a simple-to-make and delicious-to-eat topping to any of your favorite desserts!

INGREDIENTS | MAKES 2 CUPS/ 8 SERVINGS

2 15-ounce cans coconut milk
1½ tablespoons agave nectar
1½ tablespoons vanilla extract

Yes, You Can Still Enjoy Whipped Cream!

Clean eating is all about living healthier, not about deprivation. By using healthy natural ingredients to create more nutritious versions of your favorite foods, you can still indulge while actually being health-focused. There's nothing wrong with a little indulgence here and there.

1. In a stainless steel mixing bowl, combine the coconut milk, agave, and vanilla.

2. Using a high-speed handheld blender, whip the ingredients until thickened.

3. Refrigerate overnight.

PER SERVING Calories: 218.93 | Fat: 22.40 g | Protein: 2.13 g | Sodium: 13.81 mg | Fiber: 0.00 g | Carbohydrates: 6.22 g | Sugar: 3.26 g

Sweet Fruit Bake

This is a great fruit combination that—when mixed with the lemon juice—can be presented at any time without fear of it turning brown and not-so-appetizing.

INGREDIENTS | SERVES 8

2 cups blueberries, washed
2 cups strawberries, quartered
2 cups sliced peaches
2 cups sliced pears
1 tablespoon freshly squeezed lemon juice
2 tablespoons agave nectar
1 teaspoon freshly grated lemon zest

How to Grate a Lemon

To grate citrus first scrub the skin vigorously. Then, use a fine grater or Microplane to scrape the peel over a bowl. Do not grate down to where the peel begins to turn white; it's quite bitter.

1. Preheat oven to 350°F, and prepare a 9" x 13" baking dish with olive oil spray.

2. In a mixing bowl, toss all of the fruit together with the lemon juice, agave, and lemon zest.

3. Pour the fruit into the baking dish, and bake at 350°F for 25–35 minutes, or until all fruit is tender.

PER SERVING Calories: 84.59 | Fat: 0.38 g | Protein: 1.03 g | Sodium: 1.70 mg | Fiber: 3.30 g | Carbohydrates: 21.75 g | Sugar: 16.52 g

Blueberry Almond Crumble

Light and irresistible, this ooey-gooey crunchy treat is a great stand-in for butter-laden versions.

INGREDIENTS | SERVES 2

4 tablespoons filtered water

2 tablespoons agave nectar

2 pints blueberries, washed

2 tablespoons coconut oil

1 cup crushed almonds

½ cup "Good Gracious!" Granola (see recipe in Chapter 4)

Combining Antioxidants and Healthy Fats for Optimum Health

While phytonutrients and polyphenols like anthocyanins (the scientific term for the strong chemicals that make the deep colors of healthy fruit) are warriors that work wonders in the battle for a youthful, healthy, happy existence, there are elements in the diet that can actually improve their absorption and use by the body. Healthy fats like rich omegas help the body to digest and absorb fibrous fruits and veggies that contain important nutrients. By using omega-rich foods like nuts, fish, and oils, combined with these antioxidant-rich foods, we end up getting more out of every bite of the delicious and nutritious morsels we already enjoy.

1. In a small pot, combine the water and agave over medium heat, stir, and bring to a boil.

2. Reduce heat to low, add blueberries to the pot, and simmer for about 2–4 minutes (stirring constantly).

3. Pour the blueberries evenly into two medium soufflé cups, and allow to thicken.

4. Return the same pot to the medium heat and melt the coconut oil.

5. Add the almonds and granola to the coconut oil, and mix well.

6. Top the blueberries with the almonds and granola, and chill.

PER SERVING Calories: 775.62 | Fat: 45.39 g | Protein: 16.86 g | Sodium: 12.80 mg | Fiber: 15.69 g | Carbohydrates: 86.88 g | Sugar: 54.83 g

Carrot Cake

Regular carrot cake can be a delicious dessert, but can do a number on your clean-eating lifestyle. Yet it has such great potential! This cleaned-up version highlights the star of the cake— carrots—with spices—not butter and white sugar—to bring out flavor.

INGREDIENTS | SERVES 10

2 cups 100% whole wheat flour

2 teaspoons baking soda

2 teaspoons baking powder

2 teaspoons cinnamon

¼ teaspoon nutmeg

1 teaspoon all-natural sea salt

2 cups grated carrots

½ cup storebought carrot purée

1 cup vanilla almond milk

½ cup Sucanat

1½ cups unsweetened applesauce

2 teaspoons pure vanilla extract

½ cup agave nectar

½ cup crushed walnuts

1. Preheat oven to 350°F. Spray a loaf pan with olive oil spray and cover with a thin coating of wheat flour.

2. In a large mixing bowl, combine flour, baking soda, baking powder, cinnamon, nutmeg, and salt. Mix well. In a small bowl, combine the grated carrots, carrot purée, almond milk, Sucanat, applesauce, vanilla, and agave nectar and mix well.

3. Add the carrot combination to the dry ingredients, and blend well. Add walnuts and mix in thoroughly.

4. Pour the batter into the bread pan. Bake for 30–45 minutes, or until a knife inserted in the center comes out clean. Feel free to top with the delicious Clean Whipped Cream (see recipe in this chapter)!

PER SERVING Calories: 207.53 | Fat: 4.40 g | Protein: 4.71 g | Sodium: 626.54 mg | Fiber: 4.92 g | Carbohydrates: 39.98 g | Sugar: 19.14 g

Taste the Rainbow

If a food is naturally bright and colorful, it usually means that it's particularly loaded with nutrients. Bright fruits and vegetables contribute different amounts of various vitamins and minerals to our diet, which is why it's so important to vary the color experience at each meal. Red peppers, green spinach leaves, purple eggplant, orange carrots, and yellow squash all contribute something different to our body, so spread the love and taste the rainbow.

Carob Chip Walnut Cookies

Treat your sweet tooth with these clean cookies packed with healthy carob chips and natural walnuts on those special days when you deserve a deliciously sweet treat.

INGREDIENTS | MAKES 24 COOKIES

1 cup 100% whole wheat flour

1 cup oat flour

1 teaspoon baking soda

1 teaspoon baking powder

¾ cup unsweetened applesauce

½ cup Sucanat

¾ cup all-natural, organic honey

2 teaspoons pure vanilla extract

1 cup unsweetened carob chips

1 cup crushed natural walnuts

Carob Chips: A Great Alternative to Chocolate

With many recipes that contain chocolate chips having higher sugar and caffeine content than you'd want for your clean lifestyle, a simple swap for carob chips can make for a more nutritious recipe instead. Carob chips provide the same smooth texture with a hint of chocolaty-type goodness without all of the unnecessary processing and added sugars and caffeine. One great switch for healthy deliciousness!

1. Preheat oven to 350°F and prepare a baking sheet with aluminum foil and olive oil spray.

2. In a large mixing bowl, combine the flours, baking soda, and baking powder, and blend well.

3. Add the applesauce, Sucanat, honey, and vanilla to the dry ingredients, and mix to combine.

4. Fold in the carob chips and walnuts.

5. Drop the cookie mix onto the baking sheet in rounded heaping teaspoons.

6. Bake for 10–15 minutes, or until golden brown.

PER SERVING Calories: 140.59 | Fat: 4.13 g | Protein: 2.84 g | Sodium: 75.87 mg | Fiber: 1.65 g | Carbohydrates: 20.12 g | Sugar: 14.35 g

Almond Butter Cookies

These sweet cookies make for a delicious and nutritious alternative to the traditional peanut butter cookies. Just like peanut butter cookies, they're protein-packed and a favorite with kids!

INGREDIENTS | MAKES 24 COOKIES

1 cup 100% whole wheat flour
1 cup oat flour
1 teaspoon baking powder
1 cup natural almond butter
¼ cup unsweetened applesauce
1 cup honey
1 egg

Nut Butter Buyers Beware!

When purchasing a nut butter, pay close attention to the ingredients and nutrition facts. While the label may say "organic," "natural," or use other buzzwords to capture your attention, that doesn't mean you can skip reading the nutrition panel. Look for a good amount (approximately 10 g) of protein per serving with low sodium (less than 60 mg) and low sugar (less than 10 g) counts. You should not find "partially hydrogenated oils" which are also known as trans fats, in the ingredient list. Be an informed consumer!

1. Preheat oven to 350°F and prepare a baking sheet with aluminum foil and olive oil spray.

2. In a large mixing bowl, combine the flours and baking powder, and blend well.

3. Add the almond butter, applesauce, honey, and egg to the dry ingredients, and mix to combine.

4. Drop the cookie mix onto the baking sheet in rounded heaping teaspoons.

5. Bake for 10–15 minutes, or until golden brown.

PER SERVING Calories: 145.06 | Fat: 3.78 g | Protein: 3.21 g | Sodium: 26.72 mg | Fiber: 1.73 g | Carbohydrates: 26.28 g | Sugar: 15.38 g

Best-Ever Cocoa Caffe Brownies

If you're a chocolate lover who really wants to eat clean, but also has to have your occasional chocolate fix, this recipe is for you! The added plus: If you love coffee, you'll love every last bite of these delicious brownie bars!

INGREDIENTS | SERVES 9

4 squares of unsweetened dark baking chocolate, about ¾ cup

½ cup strong black coffee

½ cup unsweetened applesauce

1 tablespoon agave nectar

½ cup Sucanet

3 eggs

1 teaspoon vanilla extract

⅓ cup cocoa powder

½ cup 100% whole wheat flour

1 teaspoon baking powder

1. Preheat oven to 350°F and prepare a 9" x 9" baking pan with olive oil spray.

2. Melt the chocolate squares and set aside.

3. In a mixing bowl, combine the coffee, applesauce, agave, Sucanet, eggs, and vanilla, and mix well. Add the chocolate to the wet ingredient mixture, and mix well to combine thoroughly.

4. In a separate mixing bowl, combine the cocoa powder, flour, and baking powder, mix well, and add to the wet ingredients and combine thoroughly.

5. Pour the batter into the prepared baking dish and bake for 30 minutes, or until a fork inserted in the center comes out clean.

PER SERVING Calories: 121.656 | Fat: 7.985 g | Protein: 5.082 g | Sodium: 27.341 mg | Fiber: 3.851 g | Carbohydrates: 13.562 g | Sugar: 3.518 g

Sweet Potato Casserole with Walnut Topping

That's right, carrot cake isn't the only way to serve veggies as a dessert!

INGREDIENTS | SERVES 10

3 large sweet potatoes, peeled and cubed

1½ cups vanilla almond milk

2 eggs

1 teaspoon pure vanilla extract

1 teaspoon cinnamon

1 teaspoon cloves

½ cup Sucanat, divided

1 teaspoon ginger

2 cups crushed walnuts

½ cup coconut oil

1. In a large pot over medium heat, boil sweet potato cubes until soft.

2. Prepare a 9" x 13" baking dish with olive oil spray, and preheat oven to 400°F.

3. Drain the sweet potatoes, and mash completely. Add the almond milk, eggs, vanilla, cinnamon, cloves, ¼ cup of the Sucanat, and ginger, and blend well.

4. Pour the sweet potato mixture into the prepared baking dish.

5. In a small bowl, combine the walnuts, remaining ¼ cup of Sucanat, and coconut oil and blend well. Sprinkle the walnut mixture over the sweet potato, and bake for 35–45 minutes, or until the top is golden brown.

PER SERVING Calories: 348.38 | Fat: 27.23 g | Protein: 5.62 g | Sodium: 64.57 mg | Fiber: 3.11 g | Carbohydrates: 11.63 g | Sugar: 13.59 g

Fruity Bread Pudding

Stale bread never tasted as good as it does in this dish, absorbing the plentiful fruit juice. Vanilla almond milk makes the bread sweet and soft!

INGREDIENTS | SERVES 10

1 loaf stale whole grain, 100% whole wheat bread (torn into cubes)

2 cups strawberries, tops removed and halved

2 cups blueberries, washed

2 cups mangoes, cubed

2 cups vanilla almond milk

4 tablespoons freshly squeezed orange juice

1 tablespoon pure vanilla extract

¼ cup unsweetened applesauce

4 eggs

2 egg whites

1 teaspoon cinnamon

1 teaspoon nutmeg

Hidden Sugar Everywhere

It seems like sugar and salt are present in almost every food on grocery shelves. Whether you're trying to find a tasty salad dressing, a great stock, or a delicious chicken breast, many products are treated with added flavorings that include sugar and sodium. Even products as simple as applesauce can be sugar traps; it is of the utmost importance to pay attention to the amount of sugar, if any, in products you buy. You can always sweeten your concoctions with honey, agave, and other natural sweeteners.

1. Prepare a 9" x 13" baking dish with olive oil spray.

2. In a large mixing bowl, combine the bread and fruit, mix well, and place in the prepared baking dish.

3. In a mixing bowl, combine the almond milk, orange juice, vanilla, applesauce, eggs, and egg whites, and beat together to blend well.

4. Pour the liquid mixture over the bread and fruit and sprinkle with the cinnamon and nutmeg. Cover, refrigerate, and let the bread absorb the liquid overnight. Remove from the refrigerator 1 hour before baking.

5. Preheat oven to 350°F, and bake for 35–45 minutes or until the pudding is firm and lightly browned.

PER SERVING Calories: 355.62 | Fat: 4.02 g | Protein: 14.6 g | Sodium: 660.18 mg | Fiber: 4.49 g | Carbohydrates: 64.43 g | Sugar: 12.69 g

Maple Cinnamon Walnut Bread Pudding

When you're craving a cinnamon bun, try this clean treat instead! It's got many of the same flavors, but none of the butter and white sugar of the mall-store fat trap.

INGREDIENTS | SERVES 10

1 loaf stale whole grain, 100% whole wheat bread (torn into cubes)

1½ cups vanilla almond milk

1 tablespoon cinnamon

1 tablespoon pure vanilla extract

½ cup pure maple syrup

¼ cup unsweetened applesauce

4 eggs

2 egg whites

1 cup crushed natural walnuts

1 teaspoon nutmeg

Is Maple Syrup Good for You?

The traditional pancake syrup you probably grew up with is not natural maple syrup. When you need that specific taste for a recipe, sometimes you just have to use maple syrup. If you do, look for all-natural, organic maple syrup—it's the only product actually retrieved from maple trees and left unprocessed. The sugar content in this maple syrup is what's naturally occurring, rather than the chemically altered and manufactured version.

1. Prepare a 9" x 13" baking dish with olive oil spray.

2. Place the bread cubes in the prepared baking dish.

3. In a mixing bowl, combine the almond milk, cinnamon, vanilla, maple syrup, applesauce, eggs, and egg whites, and beat together to blend well.

4. Pour the liquid mixture over the bread cubes and sprinkle walnuts throughout; cover, refrigerate, and let the bread absorb the liquid overnight. Remove from the refrigerator 1 hour before baking.

5. Preheat oven to 350°F, sprinkle the nutmeg over top, and bake for 35–45 minutes or until the pudding is firm and lightly browned.

PER SERVING Calories: 424.46 | Fat: 11.40 g | Protein: 15.75 g | Sodium: 650.38 mg | Fiber: 3.56 g | Carbohydrates: 64.70 g | Sugar: 13.20 g

Apple Crumble

This is a yummy twist on a traditional apple streusel recipe. The delicious baked apples tossed in sweet sugar and cinnamon make every bite out of this world, but the topping makes it even better! The crunchy granola is the perfect finishing touch to the smooth apples.

INGREDIENTS | SERVES 2

4 cups Granny Smith apples, cored, peeled, and thinly sliced

¼ cup Sucanat

1 tablespoon cinnamon

½ cup crushed almonds

½ cup "Good Gracious!" Granola (see recipe in Chapter 4)

2 tablespoons coconut oil

Apples and Cinnamon for Appetite Suppressants

If you're in need of a sweet treat, but also don't want to consume an entire pie or cake, a delicious combination of apples and cinnamon may be the perfect solution. Because of the naturally occurring complex carbohydrates and fiber of apples, you achieve a feeling of fullness with much less than other foods. The cinnamon also adds a certain flavor that signals the brain and body to feel satiated. Apples and cinnamon may be the greatest combination ever!

1. Prepare a 9" x 13" baking dish with olive oil spray, and preheat oven to 375°F.

2. In a large mixing bowl, combine the apple slices, Sucanat, and cinnamon, and toss to coat. Pour the apples evenly into the prepared baking dish.

3. Combine the almonds, granola, and coconut oil together in a mixing bowl, and combine well. Crumble over top of the apples.

4. Bake for 35–45 minutes, or until topping is golden brown.

PER SERVING Calories: 722.79 | Fat: 34.14 g | Protein: 10.29 g | Sodium: 124.06 mg | Fiber: 11.12 g | Carbohydrates: 76.02 g | Sugar: 61.52 g

Cranberry Walnut Cookies

Perfect for a homemade treat you can individually freeze and enjoy anytime, or for the perfect star at a bake sale or get-together, these cookies are a great recipe you're sure to enjoy!

INGREDIENTS | SERVES 24 COOKIES

½ cup canola oil

½ cup Sucanat

1 teaspoon pure vanilla extract

1 egg

¼ cup filtered water

1 cup old-fashioned oatmeal

⅔ cup 100% whole wheat flour

1 cup unsweetened dried cranberries

1 cup crushed walnuts

½ teaspoon baking soda

½ teaspoon baking powder

Dash of all-natural sea salt

Dried Cranberries: Sweetened vs. Unsweetened

When you have a craving for dried fruits, make sure you reach for the unsweetened variety. While just ⅓ cup of dried cranberries and other dried fruits constitutes an entire fruit serving, the amount of sugar in each serving can be overwhelming. Sweetening dried cranberries with additional sugars intensifies the sweetness, but adds unnecessary sugar and carbohydrates to an otherwise perfectly healthy food.

1. Preheat oven to 350°F and prepare a baking sheet with aluminum foil and olive oil spray.

2. In a large mixing bowl, whisk together the canola oil, Sucanat, vanilla extract, egg, and water until thoroughly blended.

3. Add the oats, flour, dried cranberries, walnuts, baking soda, baking powder, and salt, and mix well.

4. Spoon the batter onto the prepared baking sheet by rounded spoonfuls, and bake for 10–15 minutes, or until golden brown.

PER SERVING Calories: 132.73 | Fat: 8.23 g | Protein: 1.91 g | Sodium: 46.46 mg | Fiber: 1.36 g | Carbohydrates: 9.60 g | Sugar: 8.16 g

Maple Rice Pudding with Walnuts

This is the absolute best rice pudding recipe out there! Not only is it a beautiful dish that's packed with the amazing flavors of maple syrup and vanilla with the added crunch of natural walnuts, it's completely clean.

INGREDIENTS | SERVES 12

3 cups uncooked brown rice

7 cups vanilla almond milk

¼ cup Sucanat

1 teaspoon vanilla extract

2 teaspoons cinnamon, divided

2 teaspoons nutmeg, divided

½ cup pure organic maple syrup

1 cup crushed walnuts

1. Preheat the oven to 325°F, and prepare a 9" x 13" casserole dish with olive oil spray.

2. In a large mixing bowl, combine the rice, almond milk, Sucanat, vanilla, 1 teaspoon of the cinnamon, and 1 teaspoon of the nutmeg. Mix well to combine.

3. Pour the mixture into the prepared baking dish, drizzle with the maple syrup, and sprinkle the walnuts and remaining cinnamon and nutmeg evenly over the top.

4. Bake for 2 hours, stirring occasionally and folding in the walnuts.

PER SERVING Calories: 226.86 | Fat: 7.98 g | Protein: 3.13 g | Sodium: 83.33 mg | Fiber: 0.96 g | Carbohydrates: 32.18 g | Sugar: 21.23 g

Clean Dream Pie Crust

Forget the storebought pie crusts! This is a simple and quick, no-bake pie crust that's crunchy and delicious. Use it for the other pies in this chapter!

INGREDIENTS | MAKES 1 PIE CRUST

4 cups macadamia nuts
1 cup coconut oil
5 dates, pitted

Homemade No-Bake Pie Crust

When was the last time you enjoyed a pie crust that had no butter, sugar, or other unhealthy oils or ingredients? Probably never. Instead, make a healthy pie crust from natural ingredients, delicious fruits, and healthy oils. Fast, easy, and delicious . . . what more could you ask for?

1. Prepare a pie dish with olive oil spray.

2. Combine all ingredients in a food processor and process until smooth.

3. Spoon the mixture into the pie pan, and press to ¼" thickness.

PER SERVING Calories: 5892.63 | Fat: 624.29 g | Protein: 43.41 g | Sodium: 27.63 mg | Fiber: 49.42 g | Carbohydrates: 105.21 g | Sugar: 50.79 g

Blueberry Pie

Scrumptious blueberry pie gets a clean makeover in this recipe. Skip the sugar and let the sweetness of the blueberries speak for itself!

INGREDIENTS | SERVES 8

3 dates, pitted
⅔ cup coconut milk
3 cups blueberries, washed
1 prepared Clean Dream Pie Crust (see recipe in this chapter)

1. In a blender, combine the dates and coconut milk, and blend until emulsified and thickened.

2. In a small pot over medium heat, bring the coconut milk and date mix to a boil. Reduce heat, add blueberries, and simmer for 5 minutes.

3. Remove the blueberries from the heat, and allow to cool for 5–10 minutes.

4. Pour the blueberries into the prepared pie shell, refrigerate, and allow to set for 3–5 hours, or overnight.

PER SERVING Calories: 158.63 | Fat: 8.84 g | Protein: 1.96 g | Sodium: 75.66 mg | Fiber: 2.03 g | Carbohydrates: 19.54 g | Sugar: 7.5 g

Cherry Pie

Guilt-free cherry pie has arrived! Creating a healthy alternative to the traditionally sugar-packed version is quick and easy with this recipe. Topped with whipped cream, granola, or left by itself, this is one beautiful pie with none of the junk ingredients!

INGREDIENTS | SERVES 8

3 dates, pitted
⅔ cup coconut milk
1 tablespoon of Sucanat
3 cups cherries, pitted
1 prepared Clean Dream Pie Crust (see recipe in this chapter)

1. In a blender, combine the dates and coconut milk, and blend until emulsified and thickened.

2. In a small pot over medium heat, bring the coconut milk and date mix to a boil. Reduce heat, add the Sucanat and cherries, and simmer for 5 minutes.

3. Remove the cherries from the heat, and allow to cool for 5–10 minutes.

4. Pour the cherries into the prepared pie shell, refrigerate, and allow to set for 3–5 hours, or overnight.

PER SERVING Calories: 169.94 | Fat: 8.77 g | Protein: 2.16 g | Sodium: 75.11 mg | Fiber: 1.91 g | Carbohydrates: 20.74 g | Sugar: 11.12 g

Apple Pie

The classic American favorite gets even better with fresh ingredients. Simple to make, and a pleasure to enjoy, this recipe provides a beautiful centerpiece for a dinner table or just the kitchen counter. Enjoy it while you can, because this pie will disappear as quickly as you made it!

INGREDIENTS | SERVES 8

4 Granny Smith apples, peeled, cored and sliced to about ⅛"
½ cup Sucanat
2 teaspoons cinnamon
1 prepared Clean Dream Pie Crust (see recipe in this chapter)

1. Toss apples in a mixing bowl with the Sucanat and the cinnamon until evenly coated.

2. Preheat oven to 400°F, and pour the apples into the prepared pie crust.

3. Bake for 35–45 minutes, or until cooked through.

4. Top with Clean Whipped Cream (see recipe in this chapter) if desired.

PER SERVING Calories: 173.66 | Fat: 4.74 g | Protein: 1.33 g | Sodium: 72.65 mg | Fiber: 1.79 g | Carbohydrates: 19.36 g | Sugar: 22.14

Coconut Cream Pie

With clean ingredients like those used to create the Clean Whipped Cream, and the Sucanat used as a more natural sweetener than table sugar, this dessert is one you can enjoy without guilt!

INGREDIENTS | SERVES 8

4 cups prepared Clean Whipped Cream (see recipe in this chapter)

½ cup Sucanat

2 cups plus 4 tablespoons unsweetened coconut flakes

1 prepared Clean Dream Pie Crust (see recipe in this chapter)

1. In a large bowl, mix the Clean Whipped Cream and the Sucanat until well-blended. Fold in 2 cups of the coconut flakes.

2. Sprinkle 2 tablespoons of the coconut flakes over the bottom of the prepared pie crust. Pour the coconut and whipped cream mixture into the pie shell, smooth the top, and sprinkle the remaining coconut flakes on top.

3. Refrigerate and chill for at least 2–4 hours, but best overnight.

PER SERVING Calories: 563.67 | Fat: 49.25 g | Protein: 4.45 g | Sodium: 117.90 mg | Fiber: 2.50 g | Carbohydrates: 15.61 g | Sugar: 15.53 g

Peach Tart

When peaches are in season, this dessert is a must-make.

INGREDIENTS | SERVES 8

4 cups peaches, peeled and sliced

¼ cup Sucanat

1 tablespoon freshly squeezed lemon juice

2 cups prepared Clean Whipped Cream, optional (see recipe in this chapter)

1 prepared Clean Dream Pie Crust (see recipe in this chapter)

1. In a mixing bowl, combine the peaches, Sucanat, and lemon juice, and toss to coat.

2. Pour the peaches into the prepared pie shell, refrigerate, and allow to set for about 3–5 hours, or overnight.

3. Cover with 2 cups of Clean Whipped Cream (if desired).

PER SERVING Calories: 313.0 | Fat: 23.37 g | Protein: 3.10 g | Sodium: 93.40 mg | Fiber: 1.61 g | Carbohydrates: 17.88 g | Sugar: 13.57 g

Frozen: The Next Best Thing

If you're making a fruit recipe, you don't *always* have to wait until the fruit you crave is in season. Manufacturers have perfected the art of flash-freezing fruits at their peak to preserve the nutrients and vitamins.

Creamy Corn Pudding

This is a sweet version of the amazingly thick and yummy traditional corn pudding. Using almond milk and Greek-style yogurt makes this dish protein-packed, and the fresh corn makes for a healthful helping of a sweet fresh vegetable packed with complex carbohydrates.

INGREDIENTS | SERVES 6

3 cups sweet corn kernels, fresh or thawed

1 cup vanilla almond milk

¼ cup plain low-fat Greek-style yogurt

2 eggs

1 tablespoon organic natural honey

¼ cup cornmeal

1 cup Cinnamon Tortilla Crisps (see recipe in Chapter 14), processed to chunky crumbs

The Truth about Corn

While it is true that corn has been taken from the fields, chemically changed, and manufactured into hundreds of thousands of products from candy bars to corn chips, the actual corn kernel is quite healthy. Packed with nutrition that's been shown to prevent illness, promote lung function, and contribute to the carbohydrate supply so important for the body's energy stores, corn is a healthy option any time.

1. Preheat the oven to 350°F and prepare a casserole dish with olive oil spray.

2. In a blender or food processor, combine half of the corn kernels, half of the almond milk, and the yogurt, and blend together until smooth.

3. In a large mixing bowl, combine the remaining almond milk, eggs, and honey, and whisk to combine thoroughly.

4. Add to the mixing bowl the processed purée, remaining corn, cornmeal, and ½ cup of the processed Cinnamon Tortilla Crisps crumbs, and mix well.

5. Pour the mixture into the casserole dish, top with remaining tortilla crumbs, and bake for 30 minutes, or until the pudding has thickened and the top is golden brown.

PER SERVING Calories: 323.47 | Fat: 12.70 g | Protein: 8.95 g | Sodium: 546.41 mg | Fiber: 3.59 g | Carbohydrates: 45.89 g | Sugar: 6.35 g

Tropical Paradise Pie

Traditional Pineapple Upside Down Cake is no competition for this delicious recipe. It's as much a visual treat as a culinary one!

INGREDIENTS | SERVES 8

3 dates, pitted

⅔ cup coconut milk

1 tablespoon of Sucanat

4 cups fresh crushed pineapple

½ cup cherries, pitted

1 prepared Clean Dream Pie Crust (see recipe in this chapter)

1. In a blender, combine the dates and coconut milk, and blend until emulsified and thickened.

2. In a small pot over medium heat, bring the coconut milk and date mix to a boil. Reduce heat, add the Sucanat, pineapple, and cherries, and simmer for 5 minutes.

3. Remove the pineapple and cherries from the heat, and allow to cool for 5–10 minutes.

4. Pour the pineapple and cherries into the prepared pie shell. Refrigerate, and allow to set for about 3–5 hours, or overnight.

PER SERVING Calories: 180.87 | Fat: 8.78 g | Protein: 2.10 g | Sodium: 75.93 mg | Fiber: 2.05 g | Carbohydrates: 23.86 g | Sugar: 13.02 g

CHAPTER 14

Clean *and* Kid-Friendly

Almond Butter Celery Sticks

Getting your kids to eat their veggies is no chore with this delicious combination. The sweetness of smooth almond butter and chewy raisins atop the crispy crunch of celery make it a noisy favorite!

INGREDIENTS | SERVES 4

4 stalks celery
½ cup almond butter
¼ cup natural unsweetened raisins

Combine Texture and Flavor

Even the pickiest of eaters normally enjoy celery topped with peanut butter. The sweet peanut butter is a tasty treat atop the crunchy, yet (let's be honest) bland-tasting celery sticks. With protein from the almond butter, rich carbohydrates, and hydrating water in the celery, it's got a plethora of nutritional benefits.

1. Clean the celery stalks by washing and cutting off the ends and tops.

2. Cut the celery sticks in half at the middle of each stalk, making 8 half-stalks.

3. Fill the center of the celery stalks with the almond butter.

4. Line the top of the almond butter with the raisins.

PER SERVING Calories: 163.73 | Fat: 7.98 g | Protein: 3.14 g | Sodium: 35.64 mg | Fiber: 2.37 g | Carbohydrates: 21.96 g | Sugar: 16.38 g

Banana Sorbet

Ice cream and storebought sorbets can be packed with sugar, fat, and impossible-to-pronounce ingredients. This recipe calls for only four ingredients, and makes for a sweet treat your kids will ask for time and time again.

INGREDIENTS | SERVES 6

4 frozen whole bananas (peeled and bagged prior to freezing)
2 teaspoons vanilla
1 teaspoon nutmeg
1 teaspoon agave nectar

Simplicity Can Be Key

When creating delicious and nutritious meals that appeal to kids, keep it simple. They may be hesitant to eat a dish that combines too many flavors—even if it's just one flavor they dislike among a ton they love. Keep it to a handful of ingredients, and add more little by little as they grow up.

1. In a high-speed blender, combine the bananas and vanilla and purée.

2. While blending, add the nutmeg and agave nectar.

3. Once fully puréed, pour the banana mixture into 6 cups, and freeze for 10 minutes.

4. Serve with a spoon.

PER SERVING Calories: 79.79 | Fat: 0.40 g | Protein: 0.89 g | Sodium: 1.03 mg | Fiber: 2.13 g | Carbohydrates: 19.31 g | Sugar: 10.88 g

Fruit Pops

Made with love and natural ingredients, these pops are healthier and more nutritious, and you're able to control the ingredients and amounts to tailor them specifically to your kids' likes and dislikes.

INGREDIENTS | SERVES 6

1 banana
1 cup strawberries, tops removed
1½ cups freshly squeezed orange juice

Frozen Delights

There's something whimsical about foods on a stick. Even adults are drawn to fair and carnival food that somehow becomes more appealing if put on a stick. Taking into consideration that kids love sweetness, sticks, and frozen treats, pops have it all wrapped up in a single delicious serving!

1. In a high-speed blender, combine the banana, strawberries, and orange juice.

2. Pour the smoothie mixture into 6 individual pop makers.

3. Freeze overnight, and remove by running the pop makers under warm water until the pops release.

PER SERVING Calories: 55.69 | Fat: 0.21 g | Protein: 0.80 g | Sodium: 1.08 mg | Fiber: 1.18 g | Carbohydrates: 13.52 g | Sugar: 8.75 g

Almond Butter and Jelly Flaxseed Roll-Ups

Sneaking in omega-rich flaxseeds is easier than ever with these scrumptious almond butter roll-ups. Perfect for healthy snacks while you watch a movie, or nutritious on-the-run munchies, these delicious roll-ups pack in flavor.

INGREDIENTS | SERVES 2

2 100% whole wheat tortillas
4 tablespoons almond butter
4 tablespoons mashed strawberries
2 tablespoons ground flaxseeds

Start Small

Almost every child has a special treat that they would eat all day, every day if they could. If you want to make that treat a little healthier, try one substitute at a time. Add a tablespoon or two of ground flaxseed to peanut butter sandwiches, peanut butter-covered brown rice cakes, or muffins to pump up your child's omega-3 intake.

1. Lay tortillas on a flat surface.

2. Spread 2 tablespoons of the almond butter on each tortilla and cover with 2 tablespoons of the mashed strawberries.

3. Sprinkle a tablespoon of the ground flaxseeds over the jelly evenly on each tortilla and roll tightly.

PER SERVING Calories: 263.93 | Fat: 12.85 g | Protein: 6.89 g | Sodium: 193.53 mg | Fiber: 4.96 g | Carbohydrates: 32.66 g | Sugar: 11.74 g

Citrus Chicken Kebobs

Because kids aren't ingrained with the "pass the salt" habit yet, these kebobs are perfect just as they are. Sweet citrus flavors the tender chicken breast on a handy kebob that's easy to eat. Remember that kids shouldn't be left unattended with sharp skewers.

INGREDIENTS | SERVES 4

2 boneless, skinless chicken breasts
1 grapefruit, inside sections removed
½ pineapple, cut into 1" cubes

Chicken: The Blank Canvas Kids Love

Packed with protein, chicken is a great low-fat food your kids can enjoy in a number of ways. Whether they prefer to have it plain, or like it more with every extra dash of spice and healthy addition, chicken is an easy-to-prepare meal for children. Lean meat like chicken can take on the flavors of anything you combine with it, which makes it a wonderful companion for delicious fresh fruit. Sweet and tangy flavors from your child's favorite fruits make each bite tender, delicious, and nutritious.

1. Cut the chicken breasts into 1" cubes, and put on a platter with the grapefruit and pineapple chunks.

2. Prepare a grill with olive oil spray to medium heat.

3. Skewer the chicken, pineapple, and grapefruit in the same rotation throughout.

4. Lay the skewers on the grill grate and grill for 5–7 minutes. Turn the skewers and continue grilling for 7 minutes, or until the chicken is completely cooked through.

5. Remove the skewers from the grill and serve.

6. **For children under seven, remove the chicken, grapefruit, and pineapple from the skewers onto a plate and serve.

PER SERVING Calories: 143.68 | Fat: 1.93 g | Protein: 13.0 g | Sodium: 44.25 mg | Fiber: 2.29 g | Carbohydrates: 20.01 g | Sugar: 15.61 g

Sweet Potato Fries

Most kids love fries. But the restaurant or takeout versions are fried in unhealthy oils and then doused in salt. Try this easy variation for a much more nutritious—but still crunchy and salty—snack.

INGREDIENTS | SERVES 4

2 sweet potatoes (peeled or with skin intact)

1 tablespoon olive oil

1 teaspoon all-natural sea salt

Health Benefits of Sweet Potatoes for Children

Rich in vitamins and minerals that remedy vitamin D deficiencies, promote healthy eyesight, and prevent illnesses like asthma by strengthening the lungs, sweet potatoes may end up being your child's favorite veggie. Sweet and versatile, there's sure to be at least one way to cook a sweet potato that will appeal to your child.

1. Preheat an oven to 400°F, and line a baking sheet with aluminum foil and olive oil spray.

2. Cut the sweet potatoes into 2"–3" long strips about ¼" in width.

3. Pour the sweet potatoes and olive oil into a large resealable plastic bag, and toss to coat.

4. Line the sweet potatoes on the baking sheet, sprinkle with half of the salt, and bake for 15–20 minutes, or until slightly crisp.

5. Flip the fries, sprinkle the remaining salt, and continue baking for 15–20 minutes, or until crispy and fork-tender.

PER SERVING Calories: 85.74 | Fat: 3.41 g | Protein: 1.02 g | Sodium: 625.62 mg | Fiber: 1.95 g | Carbohydrates: 13.08 g | Sugar: 2.72 g

Perfectly Sweet Oatmeal

Rather than loading up the day's most important meal with fat, calories, sugar, and who-knows-what-else, you can make this delicious treat in minutes with all-natural ingredients that will fuel your kids' day in the absolute best way!

INGREDIENTS | SERVES 2

2 cups rolled oats
2 cups vanilla almond milk
1 tablespoon all-natural organic maple syrup

1. Pour 1 cup of the rolled oats into each of two bowls.

2. Mix in 1 cup of almond milk and ½ tablespoon of maple syrup in each bowl.

3. Microwave on high for 2–3 minutes, or until the oats have completely absorbed all of the almond milk.

4. Stir to combine, allow to cool, and serve.

PER SERVING Calories: 417. 25 | Fat: 7.64 g | Protein: 11.59 g | Sodium: 145.77 mg | Fiber: 8.18 g | Carbohydrates: 76.52 g | Sugar: 20.79 g

Fruit Kebobs

Kebobs are just plain fun! When your kids need a snack and are bored, give them this snack/activity to keep them full—and entertained!

INGREDIENTS | SERVES 4

1 cup green seedless grapes
1 cup pineapple chunks
1 cup halved strawberries
1 cup red seedless grapes
1 cup blueberries

1. Prepare a platter with all of the fruit, and start skewers with a green grape, a pineapple chunk, a strawberry half, a red grape, and a blueberry or two.

2. Continue skewering fruit and condense firmly.

3. Serve skewers.

4. **For children under seven, remove fruit from skewers, and serve as a fruit salad instead.

PER SERVING Calories: 105.33 | Fat: 0.4 g | Protein: 1.28 g | Sodium: 2.65 mg | Fiber: 2.86 g | Carbohydrates: 27.20 g | Sugar: 21.20 g

Peanut Butter Granola Balls

These yummy treats are packed with clean carbohydrates and loads of excellent protein and omegas. You may find that they disappear awfully fast. . . .

INGREDIENTS | SERVES 5

1 cup all-natural peanut butter

2 tablespoons all-natural organic honey

2 cups "Good Gracious!" Granola (see recipe in Chapter 4)

2 tablespoons ground flaxseed

Peanut Butter and Granola for Greatness

What could be better than protein and carbohydrates that will fuel and repair your child's body for healthy activity? Peanut butter granola balls contain protein, carbohydrates, and clean healthy fats, all rolled up, literally, into great balls of goodness.

1. In a large mixing bowl, combine the peanut butter and honey, and mix until fully combined and smooth.

2. Add the granola and ground flaxseed, and stir to combine thoroughly.

3. Form the mixture into ¾"–1" balls and line up in a storage container.

4. Refrigerate for 1 hour, and serve.

PER SERVING Calories: 581.65 | Fat: 38.78 g | Protein: 20.91 g | Sodium: 249.38 mg | Fiber: 8.43 g | Carbohydrates: 43.99 g | Sugar: 21.48 g

Chicken, Rice, and Veggie Roll-Ups

When you need a change from a boring sandwich, try this filling and nutritious roll-up. It's great when you're in a hurry to get the kids off to sports practice, a theater production, or a playdate!

INGREDIENTS | SERVES 4

4 100% whole wheat tortillas

4 tablespoon plain nonfat yogurt

1 cup cooked brown rice

1 cup cooked chicken, torn into bite-sized pieces

1 cup chopped tomato

1 cup chopped romaine lettuce

Taste Vacations

If your child is open to trying new foods, try going on "taste vacations" and make Asian, Mediterranean, Thai, Italian, or African recipes.

1. Lay tortillas on a flat surface and spread 1 tablespoon of nonfat yogurt on each.

2. In a large mixing bowl, combine the rice, chicken, tomatoes, and lettuce, and spoon ¼ of the mixture down the center of each tortilla.

3. Fold in the ends, and wrap tightly.

PER SERVING Calories: 233.76 | Fat: 5.93 g | Protein: 14.76 g | Sodium: 231.45 mg | Fiber: 2.60 g | Carbohydrates: 29.73 g | Sugar: 2.61 g

Peanut Butter and Jelly Bars

Granola bars from one end of the nutritional scale to the other abound at grocery stores. This is another instance where making the item at home is much healthier. Easily stored in your freezer (but, most likely not for long!), these bars are a great snack!

INGREDIENTS | MAKES 16 BARS

3 cups all-natural peanut butter

¼ cup coconut oil

½ cup agave nectar

4 cups rolled oats

2 cups mashed strawberries

Ditch the Store-Bought Jelly

Although many jellies and jams claim to be healthy, sugar-free, and whatever else may appeal to consumers, there is no comparison between the nutrition in store-bought jellies and those made at home with natural ingredients. By creating jelly from scratch using fresh berries or other fruits you can handpick with the kiddies at local farms—mashed or puréed, sweetened with natural sweeteners or nothing at all—homemade jelly has no poor ingredients to speak of and can be enjoyed in a wide variety of ways with a million different dishes. Inexpensive, easy, and delicious, your own jelly will be the best you've ever had . . . and the most fun your kids will ever have making their own!

1. Prepare a medium saucepan with olive oil spray over medium heat, and combine 2 cups of the peanut butter, the coconut oil, and the agave nectar. Stirring constantly, mix until well-blended and melted.

2. Add the oats to the mixture, and stir to combine. Once well-blended, remove from the heat.

3. Prepare a 9" x 9" baking dish with olive oil spray. Pour half of the peanut butter–oatmeal mixture into the dish and press firmly to mold the mix as an even layer on the bottom of the pan.

4. Pour the mashed fruit over the bottom layer and spread evenly.

5. Allow the fruit layer to set for about 5 minutes, and then layer the remaining peanut butter granola mix evenly over the top.

6. Refrigerate for 1 hour, or overnight for best results. Cut into 16 rectangles.

PER SERVING Calories: 429.27 | Fat: 29.16 g | Protein: 14.95 g | Sodium: 223.86 mg | Fiber: 5.33 g | Carbohydrates: 33.28 g | Sugar: 14.24 g

Almond Butter and Banana Pitas

Pita bread is great for kids—it holds their favorite ingredients in a cute little pocket. Try this yummy combination of almond butter and banana.

INGREDIENTS | SERVES 2

1 stone-ground 100% whole wheat pita
4 tablespoons almond butter
1 tablespoon agave
1 banana, peeled and sliced

1. Cut the pita in half and open the pockets.

2. Slather the inside of each pita with the almond butter and drizzle with ½ tablespoon of agave in each.

3. Evenly layer the banana slices on one side of each pita half. Tightly close and serve.

PER SERVING Calories: 261.47 | Fat: 9.23 g | Protein: 4.47 g | Sodium: 98.97 mg | Fiber: 3.38 g | Carbohydrates: 43.47 g | Sugar: 26.49 g

"Nut" Your Everyday Trail Mix

This is an easy trail mix that's simple to put together, prepackage, and have on the go. Whenever your kids need a healthy snack that will fuel their brains and their bodies for any activity, this is a sound alternative to any storebought variety.

INGREDIENTS | MAKES 4 CUPS

1 cup "Good Gracious!" Granola (see recipe in Chapter 4)
1 cup natural, unsweetened dried cranberries
½ cup unsalted roasted sunflower seeds
½ cup unsalted cashews, crushed
½ cup natural almonds, crushed
½ cup carob chips

1. In a large resealable plastic bag, combine ingredients.

2. Pour ½ cup of the mix into separate baggies for easy access and perfect portion sizing.

3. Refrigerate bags and store in the refrigerator for up to 1 week or freeze for 1 month.

PER SERVING Calories: 714.64 | Fat: 42.46 g | Protein: 18.19 g | Sodium: 185.83 mg | Fiber: 9.68 g | Carbohydrates: 73.11 g | Sugar: 29.45 g

Crunchy Lettuce Wraps

Kids like anything that looks cool and can be wrapped up . . . especially if they can do it on their own. So this recipe is a perfect one for kids of any age. Delicious, crispy, crunchy, and packed with nutritious deliciousness, these lettuce wraps are a great sandwich alternative anytime.

INGREDIENTS | SERVES 4

1 cup plain nonfat yogurt

1 cup cooked ground chicken breast

1 cup finely chopped walnuts

1 cup green seedless grapes, quartered

½ tablespoon organic honey or agave nectar

1 tablespoon ground flaxseed

4 crisp butter lettuce leaves

1. In a large mixing bowl, combine the yogurt, chicken, walnuts, grapes, honey or agave, and flaxseed. Combine thoroughly.

2. Lay the lettuce leaves out, and spoon ¼ of the mixture into the center of each leaf.

3. Wrap tightly, and serve.

PER SERVING Calories: 350.35 | Fat: 23.82 g | Protein: 20.35 g | Sodium: 63.67 mg | Fiber: 4.68 g | Carbohydrates: 20.09 g | Sugar: 13.17 g

Change Up the Recipes to Fit Your Child's Tastes

Don't be afraid to remove, add, or change items in recipes so they're more likely to appeal to your child's tastes. If you know your child will like most of the ingredients in a recipe, but a single element would make the meal a disaster, go ahead and replace that single disliked ingredient. You know your child's likes and dislikes, so use that knowledge to your advantage and do what you can to have the most nutritious foods be the ones consumed most often. Wait a few months and try the new ingredient again.

Zucchini Muffins

Lots of kids like muffins—so build off that foundation and create some with clean ingredients! Slightly sweet and packed with tons of great nutrition, each muffin is loaded with fresh ingredients that'll fuel their school day or jumpstart their afternoon.

INGREDIENTS | MAKES 12 MUFFINS

1 large zucchini, peeled
1 cup vanilla almond milk
2 eggs, beaten
½ cup all-natural organic honey
4 tablespoons canola oil
2 cups 100% whole wheat flour
1 tablespoon baking powder
1 teaspoon all-natural sea salt
1 teaspoon cinnamon
1 teaspoon pumpkin pie spice

1. Preheat oven to 375°F and prepare 12 muffin cups with liners or olive oil spray.

2. In a food processor or blender, process the zucchini until shredded. Add the almond milk, eggs, honey, and oil to the zucchini and pulse until well-blended.

3. In a large mixing bowl, combine the dry ingredients and spices and mix well.

4. Add the zucchini mixture to the dry ingredients and stir until combined.

5. Spoon the batter evenly into the prepared muffin cups, and bake for 20–25 minutes, or until a knife inserted into the center of a muffin comes out clean.

PER SERVING Calories: 178.925 | Fat: 6.185 g | Protein: 4.818 g | Sodium: 344.094 mg | Fiber: 2.861 g | Carbohydrates: 28.645 g | Sugar: 13.227 g

Cinnamon Tortilla Crisps

Satisfy your kids' sweet teeth and the need for a LOUD crunch with these delicious cinnamon chips that are easy, clean, yummy, and 100-percent healthy!

INGREDIENTS | MAKES 40 CHIPS OR 10 SERVINGS

4 100% whole wheat tortillas

2 teaspoons cinnamon

½ teaspoon salt

Healthy Chips Okay for Kiddos

If you have a hankering for some chips and dip, but want to refrain from the salty, store-bought variety of both, you can combine these clean chips with Fruit Salsa (see recipe in Chapter 4), low-fat yogurt, or agave-sweetened Greek-style yogurt to make for a great guiltless snack for adults and kids alike!

1. Tear each tortilla into 10–12 pieces.

2. Preheat oven to 350°F. Line a baking sheet with aluminum foil and spray with olive oil spray.

3. Layer the tortilla pieces evenly on the baking sheet, spray with olive oil, and sprinkle with the cinnamon and salt.

4. Bake at 350°F for 10–15 minutes, or until crispy.

PER SERVING Calories: 38.56 | Fat: 0.94 g | Protein: 1.01 g | Sodium: 194.25 mg | Fiber: 0.61 g | Carbohydrates: 6.53 g | Sugar: 0.24 g

CHAPTER 15

Holiday Delights

Thanksgiving Roasted Turkey Breast

Rather than making an entire turkey and throwing most of its weight in bones away, there's a delicious alternative in turkey breast. Smaller, consisting mostly of white meat, moist, and delicious, this is one tasty treat that sure beats fussing with the whole bird!

INGREDIENTS | SERVES 6

1 6–8 pound turkey breast

1 tablespoon olive oil

1 teaspoon all-natural sea salt

1 teaspoon freshly ground black pepper

1 tablespoon Italian seasoning

1 lemon, sliced

Turkey Cooking Times

Knowing the weight of your bird is the most important part of figuring adequate cooking time. For example, if you have a 12–14 pound turkey, unstuffed, you can figure on a time requirement of between 3¼–3¾ hours. For each additional four pounds, you would add an additional half hour to the expected cooking time. Internal temperature readings are the only true way to tell if your turkey is done prior to carving it, so be sure to have a reliable internal temperature gauge on hand.

1. Preheat oven to 325°F, and prepare a baking pan with a roasting rack on the bottom.

2. Remove the skin from the turkey breast, pat with the tablespoon of olive oil, and season with salt, pepper, and Italian seasoning.

3. Place the turkey breast breast-side up on the roasting rack, cover with the sliced lemon, and place in the middle of the oven.

4. Baste every 20 minutes, and cook for 1–2 hours (depending upon the weight), or until the internal temperature reads 165°F.

5. Remove the turkey breast and allow the juices to redistribute, about 15 minutes, before carving and serving.

PER SERVING Calories: 520.88 | Fat: 5.20 g | Protein: 110.35 g | Sodium: 612.88 mg | Fiber: 0.37 g | Carbohydrates: 1.13 g | Sugar: 0.24 g

Meaty Herb Stuffing

Meat stuffing doesn't have to be full of fat and sodium to taste great. This hearty recipe uses delicious ground turkey breast, fragrant seasonings, and fresh veggies to make for a delicious side to any holiday feast.

INGREDIENTS | SERVES 8

2 tablespoons olive oil

1 cup chopped celery

1 cup chopped yellow or white onions

1 pound of lean ground turkey breast

2 teaspoons ground sage

2 teaspoons dried rosemary

2 teaspoons dried basil

2 teaspoons all-natural sea salt

2 teaspoons freshly ground black pepper

8 slices of stale 100% whole wheat bread, torn

Homemade Is Always the Best Bet

When you find yourself planning a meal, every dish deserves equal attention. If you plan ahead, and plan smart, you can create delicious homemade fixings to go on your holiday dinner table. Make whatever you can ahead of time to free up valuable time on the holiday itself.

1. In a large skillet over medium heat, combine ½ tablespoon of the olive oil with the chopped celery and onions. Sauté for about 3–5 minutes, or until slightly softened.

2. Add the ground turkey breast to the skillet, and season with 1 teaspoon each of the sage, rosemary, basil, sea salt, and pepper. Sauté until cooked through, remove from heat, and DO NOT DRAIN.

3. In a large serving dish, toss the meat and vegetable sauté (and all of the juices that remain) with the torn bread pieces.

4. Add the remaining olive oil (if needed) and spices to the stuffing, and toss.

5. Serve hot.

PER SERVING Calories: 170.83 | Fat: 4.65 g | Protein: 16.09 g | Sodium: 800.26 mg | Fiber: 1.39 g | Carbohydrates: 15.42 g | Sugar: 2.21 g

Cranberry Walnut Stuffing

Dried cranberries and natural walnuts give this stuffing the delicious sweet flavors of fruit with a complementary crunch.

INGREDIENTS | SERVES 4

8 slices of stale 100% whole wheat bread, torn

2 tablespoons olive oil

2 teaspoons ground sage

2 teaspoons dried rosemary

2 teaspoons dried basil

2 teaspoons all-natural sea salt

2 teaspoons freshly ground black pepper

2 cups unsweetened dried cranberries

2 cups crushed natural walnuts

Getting Creative with Fresh Ingredients

Some people tend to stick to the traditional holiday staples when preparing a holiday feast, but there's no harm in thinking outside the box. Adding fresh ingredients like cranberries and walnuts to your homemade stuffing can add a surprisingly pleasant and unexpected taste. With non-traditional seasonings—and taste and texture combinations you wouldn't normally use—you can end up with a delicious side that may become a requested staple for future occasions.

1. Preheat oven to 400°F, and line a baking sheet with olive oil spray.

2. In a large mixing bowl, combine the torn bread pieces with 1 tablespoon of olive oil, and 1 teaspoon each of the sage, rosemary, basil, sea salt, and pepper. Toss the bread to coat evenly.

3. Layer the bread pieces evenly on the prepared baking dish, and toast (tossing frequently) in the oven until slightly crunchy. Remove from heat, and pour into a large serving dish.

4. Add the remaining olive oil and spices to the stuffing, and toss to coat.

5. Fold in the dried cranberries and walnuts until well combined.

6. Serve warm.

PER SERVING Calories: 766.71 | Fat: 47.50 g | Protein: 12.95 g | Sodium: 1523.17 mg | Fiber: 9.12 g | Carbohydrates: 84.32 g | Sugar: 43.09 g

Mashed Potatoes and Cauliflower

Using half potatoes and half cauliflower, the caloric content of this delicious dish is reduced considerably. The strategic blend of herbs and spices also works well to make the dish extra-flavorful.

INGREDIENTS | SERVES 6

1 pound Idaho potatoes, peeled, washed, and cubed

1 pound cauliflower florets

2 teaspoons garlic powder

1 teaspoon onion powder

1 teaspoon all-natural sea salt

1 teaspoon freshly ground black pepper

2 cups unsweetened almond milk

1 tablespoon chopped scallions

Sneak in the Nutrition

While potatoes have loads of nutrition and tons of health benefits, there are healthy alternatives that offer different nutritional value. Adding cauliflower to your pot of boiling potatoes will result in a creamy bowl of mashed delight that's not far off from the original. The added bonus to the lower calorie load of the dish is a better variety of vitamins and minerals and the same great taste.

1. In a large pot over medium heat, bring the potato cubes to a boil, reduce heat to low, and simmer for 10 minutes.

2. Add the cauliflower to the pot and simmer for an additional 10 minutes, or until the cauliflower is fork-tender.

3. Remove the pot from the heat, drain, and move the potatoes and cauliflower to a large serving bowl. Season with the garlic powder, onion powder, salt, and pepper.

4. Mash or beat the potatoes and cauliflower, adding the almond milk ¼ cup at a time until desired texture is achieved.

5. Sprinkle the scallions over top, and serve hot.

PER SERVING Calories: 89.09 | Fat: 0.31 g | Protein: 3.26 g | Sodium: 480.99 mg | Fiber: 3.87 g | Carbohydrates: 16.71 g | Sugar: 2.39 g

Clean Green Bean Casserole

Green bean casserole is traditionally made with heavy cream or condensed soup. Saving the excess fat, calories, and sodium, this recipe uses fresh green beans and flavorful ingredients to create a great casserole with crunch and creaminess combined!

INGREDIENTS | SERVES 8

1 cup white mushrooms, minced

1 tablespoon olive oil

1 cup almond milk

1 cup nonfat plain Greek-style yogurt

6 cups cooked green beans, cleaned and halved

2 teaspoons all-natural sea salt

2 teaspoons white pepper

1 teaspoon garlic powder

1 teaspoon onion powder

Fight the Urge to Add Fat

When you find yourself looking at your traditional recipes that are tried and true, hesitating to make substitutions and alterations, remember that small changes can make a big difference. In some holiday recipes, heavy cream, condensed milk, or whole milk are the main ingredients, but flavor is the goal in using each. By replacing the fattening ingredients with fresh, more nutritious ones, you can achieve the same great taste and texture without the bad factors.

1. In a skillet over medium heat, sauté the mushrooms in the olive oil until soft and cooked through. Remove from heat, place in a mixing bowl, and allow to cool for 10 minutes.

2. Add the almond milk and yogurt to the mushrooms, and stir to combine.

3. Add the green beans, salt, pepper, garlic powder, and onion powder to the cream, and combine well.

4. Preheat the oven to 400°F, and prepare a baking dish with olive oil spray.

5. Pour the green bean mixture into the prepared casserole dish, and bake for 25–35 minutes, or until bubbly.

6. Remove the dish from the oven, and allow the casserole to cool for about 15 minutes before eating.

PER SERVING Calories: 82.37 | Fat: 2.29 g | Protein: 5.59 g | Sodium: 623.43 mg | Fiber: 3.32 g | Carbohydrates: 11.70 g | Sugar: 4.63 g

Mashed Sweet Potato Heaven

Sweet potatoes don't have to be served with crunchy or candy toppings to be delicious. This is a tasty, and very nutritious, alternative to the traditional serving of buttered mashed potatoes. If you like sweet potatoes, you'll love this side!

INGREDIENTS | SERVES 8

3 large sweet potatoes, peeled and cubed

2 tablespoons agave nectar

1 teaspoon cinnamon

1 teaspoon nutmeg

1 cup vanilla almond milk

What to Do with the Leftovers

After every holiday meal, it seems like there's more food in the fridge than there was on the table. Because most people love turkey and the fixin's—but don't want to have it for breakfast, lunch, and dinner the entire week following Thanksgiving—sometimes you have to get creative with how to reuse food. Sandwiches, wraps, soups, and salads are all different ways to create healthy meals and snacks with the leftovers in your fridge. (Search this book's index by the food you have left and find a recipe that will work!)

1. In a large pot over medium heat, bring the sweet potatoes to a boil. Reduce heat to low, and simmer until fork-tender, about 30 minutes.

2. Remove the potatoes from the heat, drain, and return to the pot.

3. Add the agave, cinnamon, and nutmeg to the sweet potatoes. Mash or beat until smooth, adding the almond milk ¼ cup at a time until desired consistency is reached.

4. Pour the sweet potatoes into a serving dish, and sprinkle lightly with cinnamon just in the center of the top.

5. Serve hot.

PER SERVING Calories: 70.76 | Fat: 0.43 g | Protein: 0.93 g | Sodium: 44.60 mg | Fiber: 1.68 g | Carbohydrates: 16.41 g | Sugar: 8.23 g

Perfect Pumpkin Pie

This creamy holiday classic is a staple in almost every home . . . and now it can be a holiday staple in the homes of clean eaters, too. Top with Clean Whipped Cream (see recipe in Chapter 13) for the best possible dessert any Thanksgiving could ask for!

INGREDIENTS | SERVES 8

1 prepared Clean Dream Pie Crust (see recipe in Chapter 13)

1 15-ounce can pure puréed pumpkin

1 cup vanilla almond milk

2 tablespoons plain nonfat Greek-style yogurt

2 eggs

½ cup honey

2 tablespoons Sucanat

2 teaspoons cinnamon

½ teaspoon pumpkin pie spice

½ teaspoon ground cloves

1. Preheat oven to 375°F, and set out the prepared pie crust.

2. In a mixing bowl, combine the pumpkin purée, almond milk, yogurt, eggs, and honey, and mix well.

3. Add the Sucanat, cinnamon, pumpkin pie spice, and cloves, and mix thoroughly.

4. Pour the pie mixture into the prepared pie crust, and bake 45–60 minutes, or until center is set and a knife inserted in the center comes out clean.

PER SERVING Calories: 204.81 | Fat: 6.25 g | Protein: 3.81 g | Sodium: 111.19 mg | Fiber: 1.10 g | Carbohydrates: 32.17 g | Sugar: 23.63 g

Pies Can Be Delicious and Healthy

With canned pumpkin purée readily available at most grocery stores, it would be a little nonsensical to steam, mash, or purée your own at triple the cost and triple the time. Make sure that your canned pumpkin is pure pumpkin with no added ingredients; the ingredient list should contain one thing and one thing only: pumpkin.

Pecan Pie

Pecan pie is normally dismissed from dieter's plates at holiday gatherings because of its ingredients and nutritional content (or the lack thereof). Enter this clean version! It's so simple and extraordinarily tasty—you'll wonder why anyone ever made it any other way.

INGREDIENTS | SERVES 8

4 cups natural pecans, divided

¾ cup coconut oil

1 cup honey

1½ cups dates, pitted

1 teaspoon ground nutmeg

1 teaspoon cinnamon

1 teaspoon ground cloves

1 prepared Clean Dream Pie Crust (see recipe in Chapter 13)

Pecan Pie Gets a Clean Makeover

Pecan pie is a holiday favorite that must be avoided at all costs, right? Wrong! Pecans are an amazing source of protein and healthy fats and, combined with fresh natural ingredients, can deliver the same great taste as traditional, but not-so-healthy versions of pecan pie. Healthy, packed with benefits for the body and the brain, and amazingly delicious, this is a pie that's delicious and nutritious from the crust to the filling to the topping!

1. In a food processor, process 3 cups of the pecans, coconut oil, honey, and dates until thickened. Move to a mixing bowl, and add the nutmeg, cinnamon, and cloves to the pecan mix, and blend well.

2. Set out the prepared pie shell.

3. Pour the pecan mix into the pie shell, and top with the remaining pecans. Press them lightly into the pie, and allow the pie to set for 3–4 hours.

PER SERVING Calories: 864.44 | Fat: 64.58 g | Protein: 7.08 g | Sodium: 75.70 mg | Fiber: 8.74 g | Carbohydrates: 76.68 g | Sugar: 58.20 g

Holiday Scalloped Potatoes

At holiday time, mashed potatoes can get a little mundane and routine, so this recipe comes to the rescue at the perfect time! Again, we'll use flavorful spices and protein-rich almond milk to give the dish its flair. Healthy and delicious, even at the holidays!

INGREDIENTS | SERVES 6

6 large Idaho potatoes
2 cups unsweetened almond milk
2 cups crumbled goat cheese
1 cup scallions, chopped
2 teaspoons garlic powder
2 teaspoons onion powder
1 teaspoon freshly ground black pepper

1. With a mandoline, slice the potatoes thinly.

2. In a large mixing bowl, combine the potatoes, almond milk, goat cheese, scallions, garlic powder, onion powder, and pepper.

3. Preheat oven to 400°F, and prepare a 9" x 13" casserole dish with olive oil spray.

4. Pour the potato mixture into the casserole dish, and bake for 45–60 minutes, or until bubbly and golden brown.

5. Remove from heat, and allow to set and thicken for about 10–15 minutes before serving.

PER SERVING Calories: 508.73 | Fat: 26.89 g | Protein: 27.13 g | Sodium: 334.80 mg | Fiber: 6.03 g | Carbohydrates: 37.52 g | Sugar: 4.94 g

Better Than Classic Cranberry Sauce

This is a super-simple recipe that uses fresh ingredients and makes for a tasty cranberry sauce you'll be proud to put on your holiday table. Using only four ingredients, and prepared in only one pot, you'll save time and cleanup by going with this clean version!

INGREDIENTS | SERVES 6

1 cup freshly squeezed orange juice

¼ cup agave nectar

1 tablespoon orange zest

1 pound cranberries, washed

Cranberry Sauce for . . . Anything!

If you're wondering what to have for dinner on a random evening, don't forget about cranberry sauce recipes like this one! Topping chicken and fish, this makes for a great sweet sauce that perfectly complements a slightly salty entrée. Tossed in salads, this recipe's sauce can provide sweet flavor, smooth texture, and astounding health benefits. So, remember: Cranberry sauce isn't just for Thanksgiving!

1. In a large pot over medium heat, bring the orange juice, agave, and orange zest to a boil. Reduce the heat to low, and simmer.

2. Add the washed cranberries to the pot, and simmer for about 10–15 minutes, or until the cranberries begin to burst.

3. Remove from heat, stir, and allow the sauce to thicken.

4. Serve warm or cold.

PER SERVING Calories: 98.50 | Fat: 0.15 g | Protein: 0.63 g | Sodium: 2.89 mg | Fiber: 3.63 g | Carbohydrates: 25.76 g | Sugar: 18.24 g

Creamy Asparagus Casserole

Green beans aren't the only green veggies you can dress up for your dinner table. These deliciously crisp asparagus spears, in a creamy dressing of healthy ingredients lightly flavored with spices, makes for a light side dish that's mouthwatering and nutritious.

INGREDIENTS | SERVES 8

1 cup yellow onion, diced
1 tablespoon olive oil
1 cup unsweetened almond milk
1 cup plain nonfat Greek-style yogurt
6 cups asparagus spears, cleaned
2 teaspoons all-natural sea salt
2 teaspoons white pepper
1 teaspoon garlic powder

1. In a skillet over medium heat, sauté the onions in the olive oil until soft and cooked through. Remove from heat and place in a mixing bowl.

2. Add the almond milk and yogurt to the onions, and stir to combine.

3. Add the asparagus, salt, pepper, and garlic powder to the cream, and combine well.

4. Preheat the oven to 400°F, and prepare a 9" x 13" baking dish with olive oil spray.

5. Pour the asparagus mixture into the prepared casserole dish, and bake for 25–35 minutes, or until bubbly.

6. Remove the dish from the oven, and allow the casserole to cool for about 15 minutes before eating.

PER SERVING Calories: 69.25 | Fat: 1.84 g | Protein: 5.96 g | Sodium: 629.66 mg | Fiber: 2.76 g | Carbohydrates: 7.70 g | Sugar: 3.98 g

Delicious Prime Rib

Rather than packing a prime rib with loads of salt, you can opt for a healthier recipe that makes delicious use of spices instead. Creating healthy cuts of this beautiful roast will make for an enjoyable meal with tender meat full of flavor, not sodium.

INGREDIENTS | SERVES 12

1 tablespoon minced garlic

1 tablespoon celery seed

2 teaspoons all-natural sea salt

1 tablespoon freshly ground black pepper

2 teaspoons onion powder

14-pound prime rib roast, trimmed of the fat

2 tablespoons olive oil

How Long Does It Cook?

Delicious prime rib is a great holiday meal that's healthy and packed with tons of flavor. One great thing about prime rib is that its cuts, from the outside to the center, can fulfill any guest's desire for doneness. The outer ends may be well done with the center a beautiful medium rare. But how do you know when it's reached the perfect temperature? A handy, and very inexpensive, tool called a meat thermometer inserted into the meat will tell you the doneness of the meat in seconds. For medium rare, aim for a temp of 130–140°F, medium reads 140–150°F, and well done reads 150–165°F.

1. Preheat oven to 400°F and prepare a large roasting pan.

2. Combine the celery seed, sea salt, pepper, and onion powder in a small dish.

3. Pat the rib roast with the olive oil, pat on the minced garlic, and sprinkle the entire roast with the spice mixture.

4. Bake for 4–5 hours or until an internal temperature shows the corresponding doneness desired.

PER SERVING Calories: 1676.00 | Fat: 145.03 g | Protein: 85.17 g | Sodium: 681.74 mg | Fiber: 0.14 g | Carbohydrates: 0.76 g | Sugar: 0.04 g

Mega Mushroom Gravy

One delicious staple on any holiday table is the gravy. Once infamous for being full of fat, sodium, and empty calories, this recipe makes a delicious version full of fresh ingredients. This thick gravy gets the majority of its flavor from the mushrooms being sautéed first.

**INGREDIENTS | MAKES 4 CUPS
(16 SERVINGS)**

1 tablespoon olive oil

5 cups sliced portabella mushrooms

1 teaspoon garlic powder

1 teaspoon freshly ground black pepper

2 teaspoons all-natural sea salt

4 tablespoons oat flour

4 cups unsweetened almond milk

1. In a saucepan over medium heat, combine the olive oil, mushrooms, garlic powder, pepper, and 1 teaspoon of the sea salt. Sauté the mushrooms until they are soft and tender, about 6–8 minutes.

2. Whisk the flour and remaining teaspoon of salt into the almond milk until well blended.

3. Add the almond milk to the mushrooms gradually, ¼ cup at a time, stirring constantly. Reduce heat to low.

4. Once the sauce begins to thicken, continue to simmer for 1–2 minutes, and remove from heat. Allow to set about 5 minutes, and serve.

PER SERVING Calories: 38.43 | Fat: 1.26 g | Protein: 1.37 g | Sodium: 342.99 mg | Fiber: 0.88 g | Carbohydrates: 3.55 g | Sugar: 0.71 g

Green Beans Almondine

This is one of the healthiest holiday dishes around. Perfect for the holidays, this is a bright green dish of few ingredients that is fresh and absolutely delicious!

INGREDIENTS | SERVES 6

1 pound green beans, cleaned and trimmed

2 tablespoons extra-virgin olive oil

½ cup slivered almonds

1 teaspoon freshly squeezed lemon juice

1 teaspoon all-natural sea salt

1. In a medium saucepan, bring the green beans to a boil, reduce heat, and simmer until tender but still crisp.

2. Remove the green beans from the heat, and drain.

3. Place the green beans in a large serving dish, and toss with the olive oil, almonds, lemon juice, and sea salt until well combined.

PER SERVING Calories: 108.63 | Fat: 8.58 g | Protein: 3.05 g | Sodium: 4.83 mg | Fiber: 2.99 g | Carbohydrates: 6.98 g | Sugar: 2.77 g

Holiday Appetizers: Clean and Delicious!

Holiday appetizers can get a little tricky if you're trying to adhere to a clean lifestyle. Avoiding cheeses, high-fat creams, and unnecessary white flour and sugar, you can actually create a wide variety of delicious appetizers that will please and promote health. Homemade chips and dips, salsas, salads, and even meat and meatless entrees can be whipped up in a flash and plated to serve many . . . all clean, too!

Christmas Morning Sausage Soufflé

Christmas mornings can be pretty busy, and breakfast is the last thing you want to be tending to when there are gifts to open and pictures to take. This recipe can be made the night before and refrigerated, so your Christmas-morning duties are only to put it in the oven!

INGREDIENTS | SERVES 16

1 pound lean ground beef
2 tablespoons coriander seeds
2 teaspoons garlic powder
2 teaspoons onion powder
2 teaspoons all-natural sea salt
2 teaspoons freshly ground black pepper
1 tablespoon olive oil
1 cup onions, diced
1 cup mushrooms, diced
1 cup green pepper, diced
1 cup red pepper, diced
12 eggs
2 cups unsweetened almond milk
1 cup crumbled goat cheese

Try a Vegetarian Version!

It's simple to turn this soufflé into a vegetarian dish. Just replace the ground beef and coriander with 4 cups of hash brown potatoes! Add them when you beat the eggs, milk, and goat cheese, and voilá!

1. Preheat oven to 375°F and prepare a baking dish with olive oil spray.

2. In a large mixing bowl, combine the ground beef, coriander seeds, and 1 teaspoon each of the garlic and onion powders, salt, and pepper. Combine well.

3. In a large skillet over medium heat, warm the olive oil and sauté the onions, mushrooms, and peppers until slightly softened. Add the beef mixture to the pan, and sauté until cooked through. Remove from heat, and allow to cool for 15 minutes.

4. In the large mixing bowl, beat together the eggs, almond milk, goat cheese, and remaining spices until well combined. Add the sautéed beef and vegetables to the beaten eggs, and combine well.

5. Pour the mixture into the prepared baking dish and bake for 1 hour, or until golden brown and cooked through.

PER SERVING Calories: 181.09 | Fat: 11.14 g | Protein: 15.71 g | Sodium: 438.59 mg | Fiber: 1.06 g | Carbohydrates: 3.54 g | Sugar: 1.58 g

Savory Corn Pudding

This delicious dish is a beautiful addition to any holiday table setting. Sprinkled with delicious vegetables and spices, this is a savory variation of the sweet Creamy Corn Pudding (see recipe in Chapter 13) recipe.

INGREDIENTS | SERVES 6

2 cups sweet corn kernels, fresh or thawed

1 cup unsweetened almond milk

¼ cup plain nonfat Greek-style yogurt

2 eggs

2 teaspoons all-natural sea salt

2 teaspoons freshly ground black pepper

2 teaspoons garlic powder

1 cup scallions, chopped

1 cup chopped red bell peppers

¼ cup cornmeal

1 cup Tasty Tortilla Chips (see recipe in Chapter 4), processed to chunky crumbs

1. Preheat the oven to 350°F and prepare a 9" x 13" casserole dish with olive oil spray.

2. In a blender or food processor, combine half of the corn kernels, half of the almond milk, and the yogurt, and blend together until smooth.

3. In a large mixing bowl, combine the remaining almond milk, eggs, and spices, and whisk to combine thoroughly.

4. Add to the mixing bowl the processed purée, remaining corn, scallions, red pepper, cornmeal, and ½ cup of the processed Tasty Tortilla Chips crumbs, and mix well.

5. Pour the mixture into the casserole dish, top with remaining tortilla crumbs, and bake for 30 minutes, or until the pudding has thickened and the top is golden brown.

PER SERVING Calories: 308.18 | Fat: 12.19 g | Protein: 8.85 g | Sodium: 1254.73 mg | Fiber: 4.19 g | Carbohydrates: 41.53 g | Sugar: 4.78 g

Corn Bread

This recipe makes good use of every ingredient by making healthy substitutes for the poor ingredients of the traditional recipes. Even though the switcheroo took out the butter, sugar, and salt, you'll be amazed how delicious this corn bread became without them.

INGREDIENTS | SERVES 6

2 tablespoons 100% whole wheat flour (for coating of pan)

1 cup plain nonfat yogurt

2 tablespoons plain Greek-style yogurt

2 eggs

2 tablespoons applesauce

1 tablespoon Sucanat

2 cups kernel corn, fresh or frozen

1 cup self-rising cornmeal

1. Preheat the oven to 375°F, and coat a loaf pan with olive oil spray and whole wheat flour.

2. In a large mixing bowl, combine the yogurts, eggs, applesauce, Sucanat, and corn, and mix well.

3. Add the cornmeal gradually, and combine thoroughly.

4. Pour the mix into the prepared bread pan, and bake for 20–30 minutes, or until golden brown and a knife inserted in the center comes out clean.

PER SERVING Calories: 201.12 | Fat: 3.83 g | Protein: 7.53 g | Sodium: 49 mg | Fiber: 2.51 g | Carbohydrates: 33.87 g | Sugar: 7.50 g

Pineapple Centerpiece with Fruit Skewers

This pineapple will be the talk of the party! Making for the most beautiful (and edible) centerpiece you've ever seen, this is an easy way to display the healthiest fresh fruit in the most stylish of ways. Your guests will enjoy grabbing a skewer and having a serving of fruit right in their hand.

INGREDIENTS | SERVES 20–30

1 large pineapple
4 cups pineapple, in cubes
4 cups strawberries
1 pound green seedless grapes
1 pound red seedless grapes
4 cups clementine segments
4 cups blueberries
20–30 skewers, 10–12"

1. Place the pineapple in the center of a serving tray.

2. Skewer the fruit in the following order: pineapple, strawberries, grapes, clementines, and blueberries until all skewers are completed.

3. Stab the skewers into the pineapple with the largest fruit flush against the pineapple.

4. Rotate the pineapple, and continue adding the skewers evenly throughout the pineapple's surface until all are completely set.

PER SERVING Calories: 76.9 | Fat: 0.28 g | Protein: 0.93 g | Sodium: 1.81 mg | Fiber: 2.23 g | Carbohydrates: 19.90 g | Sugar: 15.20 g

APPENDIX A

Eating Clean Meal Plan

By using the following meal plans as a general guide, you can get an idea of the types of foods and portion sizes that could constitute a daily clean menu. Since the clean lifestyle focuses on meals and snacks that are separated by only 3–4 hours, each day's number of meals and times will vary slightly depending upon the first meal's time. For example, a day's first meal at 7:00 A.M. would be followed with meals or snacks at 10:00 A.M., 1:00 P.M., 4:00 P.M., and 7:00 P.M., making for five total servings throughout the day. (An additional meal at 10:00 P.M. would be too close to bedtime.) If you're a very early riser, a day's first meal at 4:00 A.M. would be followed by meals or snacks at 7:00 A.M., 10:00 A.M., 1:00 P.M., 4:00 P.M., and 7:00 P.M., making for six total servings throughout the day.

The caloric content of each day's meals and snacks will also vary depending upon the amount of calories required by each individual. Obviously, a large man requiring 2,500 calories per day will have different caloric needs than a petite woman requiring 1,600 calories, meaning that they should make different meal choices. Keeping these main ideas in mind while planning the day's foods will ensure that your clean lifestyle will be the most beneficial way of life for your mind and body.

Another key point to pay attention to in planning your day's meals is the amount, type, and time of activity that will be occurring around each meal and snack. Schedule a large meal consisting of mostly carbohydrates prior to an exercise session to ensure that you'll have energy for the workout; don't eat that same meal before a long session of office work or extended "downtime" where little activity is performed. If you're aware of when your activity levels are at their highest, you can more easily plan the types of foods, and amounts, that make sense for each meal and snack. Keeping a journal about these activities can be very helpful in planning the meals for the upcoming days and weeks . . . which can also simplify grocery shopping!

Remember, the clean lifestyle shouldn't be difficult, so make it easy and enjoyable by following these simple rules of thumb. Don't forget . . . Enjoy!

▼ 14-DAY MEAL PLAN

	BREAKFAST	SNACK	LUNCH	SNACK	DINNER
Day 1	Baked Apples and Cinnamon	Strawberry Dream Smoothie	Curry Chicken Gyros	Simple Spinach Salad	Fabulous Fish Tacos with Stuffed Mushrooms
Day 2	Blazing Blueberry Muffins	Grilled Tomato and Pesto Salad	Spicy Chipotle Grilled Shrimp	Savory Spinach and Garlic Smoothie	Tempeh Fajitas with Scalloped Tomatoes
Day 3	Fruity Yogurt Parfaits	Peanut Butter Granola Balls	Amazing Minestrone Soup	Melon Mix-Up	Lemon-Basil Chicken and Spicy Broccolini
Day 4	Sweet Potato Pancakes	Peaches 'n Cream Smoothie	Marvelous Mediterranean Wrap	Strawberry Walnut Flaxseed Salad	Italian Portabella Burgers with Zucchini Boats
Day 5	Cranberry Orange Bread	Tropical Paradise Smoothie	Garlic Ginger Tofu	White Bean Wonder Soup	Tomato-Basil Rigatoni
Day 6	Very Veggie Frittata	Asian Almond Mandarin Salad	Ultimate Black Bean Burgers	Perfect Pear Smoothie	Feisty Fish Tabbouleh
Day 7	Fruit-Stuffed French Toast Sandwiches	Scrumptious Salsa with Tasty Tortilla Chips	Chicken Salad Pita	Mango Madness Smoothie	Thai Coconut Chicken with Carrot Coleslaw
Day 8	Pumpkin Flaxseed Muffins	Very Cherry Vanilla Smoothie	Tuna Salad–Stuffed Tomatoes with Perfect Polenta	Creamy Asparagus Soup	Spinach-Stuffed Chicken with Broccoli-Cauliflower Bake
Day 9	Creamy Blueberry Smoothie	Spicy Eggs with Romaine and Arugula	Too-Good Turkey Burger with "Lighten Up" Potato Salad	Cream of Broccoli Soup	Balsamic Chicken with Artichokes and Fire-Roasted Tomatoes with Scalloped Potatoes with Leeks and Olives
Day 10	Pumpkin Spice Smoothie	Chicken and Apple Spinach Salad	Easy Omelet	Split Pea Soup and Stuffed Mushrooms	Shrimp Pasta Bake
Day 11	Banana Bread with Walnuts and Flaxseeds	Cucumber Salad	Grilled Chicken and Pineapple Sandwich	Cran-Orange Oatmeal	Bean Burritos and Mediterranean Couscous
Day 12	Apple-Nana Muffins	Quickie Quesadillas	Creamy Macaroni Salad	Clean Green Go-Getter Smoothie	Garlic Chicken Stir-Fry with "Not Fried" Fried Rice
Day 13	Pineapple Delight Smoothie	Honey Mustard Chicken Tenders	Roasted Red Pepper Hummus	Tomato Caprese Salad	Tuna Noodle Casserole with Classic Antipasto Salad
Day 14	All Almonds Smoothie	Roasted Red Pepper Hummus with Tasty Tortilla Chips	Shrimp Salsa Pita	Scrumptious Sage and Squash Soup	Pork Loin and Roasted Root Vegetables with Sunshine Corn Muffins

Standard U.S./Metric Measurement Conversions

VOLUME CONVERSIONS

U.S. Volume Measure	Metric Equivalent
⅛ teaspoon	0.5 milliliters
¼ teaspoon	1 milliliters
½ teaspoon	2 milliliters
1 teaspoon	5 milliliters
½ tablespoon	7 milliliters
1 tablespoon (3 teaspoons)	15 milliliters
2 tablespoons (1 fluid ounce)	30 milliliters
¼ cup (4 tablespoons)	60 milliliters
⅓ cup	90 milliliters
½ cup (4 fluid ounces)	125 milliliters
⅔ cup	160 milliliters
¾ cup (6 fluid ounces)	180 milliliters
1 cup (16 tablespoons)	250 milliliters
1 pint (2 cups)	500 milliliters
1 quart (4 cups)	1 liter (about)

WEIGHT CONVERSIONS

U.S. Weight Measure	Metric Equivalent
½ ounce	15 grams
1 ounce	30 grams
2 ounces	60 grams
3 ounces	85 grams
¼ pound (4 ounces)	115 grams
½ pound (8 ounces)	225 grams
¾ pound (12 ounces)	340 grams
1 pound (16 ounces)	454 grams

OVEN TEMPERATURE CONVERSIONS

Degrees Fahrenheit	Degrees Celsius
200 degrees F	95 degrees C
250 degrees F	120 degrees C
275 degrees F	135 degrees C
300 degrees F	150 degrees C
325 degrees F	160 degrees C
350 degrees F	180 degrees C
375 degrees F	190 degrees C
400 degrees F	205 degrees C
425 degrees F	220 degrees C
450 degrees F	230 degrees C

BAKING PAN SIZES

American	Metric
8 x 1½ inch round baking pan	20 x 4 cm cake tin
9 x 1½ inch round baking pan	23 x 3.5 cm cake tin
11 x 7 x 1½ inch baking pan	28 x 18 x 4 cm baking tin
13 x 9 x 2 inch baking pan	30 x 20 x 5 cm baking tin
2 quart rectangular baking dish	30 x 20 x 3 cm baking tin
15 x 10 x 2 inch baking pan	30 x 25 x 2 cm baking tin (Swiss roll tin)
9 inch pie plate	22 x 4 or 23 x 4 cm pie plate
7 or 8 inch springform pan	18 or 20 cm springform or loose bottom cake tin
9 x 5 x 3 inch loaf pan	23 x 13 x 7 cm or 2 lb narrow loaf or pate tin
1½ quart casserole	1.5 liter casserole
2 quart casserole	2 liter casserole

Index

Note: Page numbers in **bold** indicate recipe category lists.

We Have
EVERYTHING
on Anything!

With more than 19 million copies sold, the Everything® series has become one of America's favorite resources for solving problems, learning new skills, and organizing lives. Our brand is not only recognizable—it's also welcomed.

The series is a hand-in-hand partner for people who are ready to tackle new subjects—like you!

For more information on the Everything® series, please visit *www.adamsmedia.com*

The Everything® list spans a wide range of subjects, with more than 500 titles covering 25 different categories:

Business	History	Reference
Careers	Home Improvement	Religion
Children's Storybooks	Everything Kids	Self-Help
Computers	Languages	Sports & Fitness
Cooking	Music	Travel
Crafts and Hobbies	New Age	Wedding
Education/Schools	Parenting	Writing
Games and Puzzles	Personal Finance	
Health	Pets	